The Gluten Lie

And other myths about what you eat

Alan Levinovitz

Regan Arts.

NEW YORK

If you stopped eating gluten, you'd feel way fucking better all day. Whenever you feel shitty, that's because of gluten. It's just true. Gluten's a vague term. It's something used to categorize things that are bad. You know, calories. That's a gluten. Fat, that's a gluten.

—SETH ROGEN IN *THIS IS THE END*

The Gluten Lie

Contents

INTRODUCTION

Once Upon a Toxin

More than 100 million Americans want to avoid gluten, and they are in good company. Oprah's twenty-one-day cleansing diet is gluten-free. Bill Clinton's personal weight-loss guru, Dr. Mark Hyman, has asked if modern "super-gluten" is a dietary demon. In the best-selling book *Grain Brain*, neurologist David Perlmutter argues that it causes dementia and Alzheimer's. And in *Wheat Belly* (over 1 million copies sold), cardiologist William Davis includes a section titled, in all-caps, "BREAD IS MY CRACK!" Dietary demon, indeed.

It's hard to believe that twenty years ago virtually no one, including health enthusiasts, had even heard of gluten. Best-selling diet books omitted it entirely. Back then, the nation's latest dietary demon had a different name: monosodium glutamate.

Where menus and labels now advertise foods as "Gluten Free," restaurant owners and manufacturers once had to reassure their customers with a different promise: NO MSG. True, MSG *seems* safe—it's a sodium salt first extracted from seaweed by Japanese scientists in

1908, and a staple seasoning in the cuisine of long-lived East Asians. But health-conscious Americans knew better. Everyone had read the newspapers and watched the TV exposés, which revealed the crystalline flavor enhancer as a deadly poison. By the mid-1980s, it was common knowledge that MSG caused devastating migraines, irritable bowel syndrome, and a suite of other symptoms. Still worse, some authorities believed it caused brain damage and chronic disease. Only fools and Chinese people would risk their health by consuming such a potent toxin.

The MSG scare began on April 4, 1968, with a letter to the *New England Journal of Medicine* from Chinese American physician Robert Ho Man Kwok. In the letter, titled "Chinese-Restaurant Syndrome," Kwok reported that after eating in Chinese restaurants he regularly experienced numbness, general weakness, and palpitation. His colleagues had suggested he was allergic to soy sauce, but Kwok knew that couldn't be right. He often used soy sauce in his own home cooking with no ill effect.

"The cause is obscure," he admitted, before identifying three likely suspects: cooking wine ("because the syndrome resembles to some extent the effects of alcohol"), monosodium glutamate, and the high levels of sodium in restaurant Chinese food.

An avalanche of responses poured into the *NEJM*. Everyone had experienced the syndrome! In May, the journal printed no less than ten of these letters, many written by highly credentialed physicians, each endorsing a different cause of "Chinese restaurant syndrome." One suggested "muscarine poisoning" related to the ingestion of imported mushrooms. Another singled out "the elusive tannins of tea" and "frozen-food processing of Chinese vegetables." Terrifyingly, one neurologist recounted treating a stroke in an otherwise healthy patient—inexplicable, save for the fact that three hours earlier the man had eaten Chinese food.

The rapidity with which MSG became a nationally recognized health threat is astonishing, especially given that this was 1968, a time when telephone wires and printed paper still regulated the spread of information. Less than two months after Kwok's letter, the *New York Times* ran an article under the headline "Chinese Restaurant Syndrome Puzzles Doctors." Within six months, the prestigious journal *Nature* published research by scientists who definitively identified MSG as the culprit—and, alarmingly, pointed out that it lurked everywhere, not just in Chinese food: TV dinners, canned goods, seasoning, even baby food.

Utterly convinced by their research, the authors of the *Nature* article sought out a young lawyer-advocate named Ralph Nader, with whom they campaigned to have MSG removed from baby food and stricken from the Food and Drug Administration's Generally Recognized as Safe list. In October 1969, Gerber, Heinz, and Squibb Beech-Nut caved to enormous public pressure and announced that their baby food would no longer be made with MSG. And on April 4, 1970, two years to the day from the publication of Kwok's letter, the National Research Council ruled that MSG was "fit for human consumption but not necessarily by infants," a cryptic pronouncement that only heightened safety concerns.

For millions of sufferers, the "discovery" of MSG sensitivity came as a tremendous relief. Headaches, upset stomachs, aching joints, cold sweats, colicky babies—finally, the mystery of endless recurring ailments had been solved. And the solution made sense. Most domestic cooks were unfamiliar with monosodium glutamate, a foreign, scary-sounding chemical. Food industry spokespeople were calling for calm deliberation—proof positive they were hiding something big. After all, if there was no need for concern, why did they go ahead and remove MSG from baby food?

But amid the outcry against MSG, science marched on, ever skeptical of snap judgments and anecdotal evidence. After many rigorous studies, the panic proved unfounded. In contrast to popular belief, clinical trials strongly suggested that MSG did not produce symptoms like migraines. Today, food allergy experts believe the overwhelming majority of reactions to MSG are psychological, not physiological. According to the 2013 edition of *Food Allergy: Adverse Reactions to Foods and Food Additives,* a comprehensive reference manual for hospitals and private practitioners, there is little doubt about "the rarity of the MSG symptom complex even among individuals who believe themselves to be MSG sensitive." In other words: your MSG headaches are probably just headaches.

When it comes to food sensitivities, people are incredibly unwilling to question self-diagnoses.

But when it comes to food sensitivities, people are incredibly unwilling to question self-diagnoses. No one wants to think that the benefits they experienced from going gluten-free or eliminating MSG might be psychological. That would mean the problem was psychological to begin with, and there's something intensely disturbing about the notion that we can make ourselves sick. Psychology, not physiology, becomes the mechanism of illness, and the individual displaces bad food as the source of blame for their suffering. This can make us feel vulnerable, stupid, and weak, as though we have the choice to be better but lack the mental acuity to manage it. On top of all that, it's hard not to feel like a psychological explanation trivializes your condition—hence the expression "It's *only* in your head."

And so the myth of MSG sensitivity lives on. Among those who believe they react to MSG, the long-standing conclusion of allergists borders on heresy and often provokes extreme anger. Here are two representative responses to a 2014 online essay, "Is MSG Misunderstood?," published on Livestrong.com, a popular source of health information:

What an insensitive article. I am a person who suffers, SUFFERS, when I consume MSG. I get a terrible migraine and feel awful for hours. For me, this result is consistent and reproducible. I lived with these migraines for years before discovering what triggered them. It is very upsetting to read an article telling me that my symptoms are psychosomatic.

This is like saying the devil is good. I went to a Chinese restaurant for my son's birthday and after feasting when we came out, he as [sic] disoriented and ripped of [sic] the rearview mirror. You cannot rehabilitate MSG so just stop or I will stop reading your blog.

The anger in these comments reflects the unwavering faith people place in their own dietary diagnoses, a faith that is often misplaced. Figuring out the effects of one's diet is enormously complicated. For most of us, cutting out MSG or going gluten-free involves broader changes in how we approach food. That makes it difficult to sort out what caused what. Your headaches went away—but was it the absence of MSG or an increase in home-cooked meals? Did you lose weight by going gluten-free or by eating less fast food? To complicate matters further, discovering a dietary solution feels empowering, and empowerment itself can lead to significant positive physiological changes. Unless we can be absolutely certain of our self-diagnosis, it's best to keep an open mind about alternative explanations.

But admitting uncertainty is hard, particularly uncertainty about how our own bodies work. So instead, we lie to ourselves. We lie to ourselves about our ability to recall symptoms and their intensity—the fact of having had a headache, say, and its severity. We lie to ourselves about our ability to recall what we've eaten, a perennial problem for researchers who rely on self-reported food consumption data. (Can you really remember how much kung pao chicken you ate two weeks ago? Did you eat more of the vegetables, the chicken, or the peanuts?)

Finally, we lie to ourselves about our ability to accurately diagnose the relationship between what we consume and our experience of physical and mental symptoms.

Scientists universally acknowledge the prevalence of these lies. They are the reason for placebo-controlled studies of food and medicine—like those conducted on MSG—which substitute a neutral substance for the substance being tested. Placebo-controlled studies are necessary to distinguish actual physiological effects from the power of positive (or negative) thinking. Antidepressants—and gluten-free diets—can make us feel better just because we think they will. And MSG can make us sick for the same reason.

That's why personal testimonials cannot, in themselves, establish the efficacy of a drug or diet. Just imagine if being super-convinced that something worked made it a legitimate treatment. Blessed water from the fountain at Lourdes would count as highly effective medicine. Exorcism would be a great way to deal with behavioral problems. And modern medical science as we know it wouldn't exist.

Everyone recognizes that expectations can shape experiences and distort memories. Yet while most of us recognize how self-deception shapes stories about supernatural healing, we are less willing to consider how it might shape our own stories of dietary salvation.

Unfortunately, where people are prone to self-deception, they are also open to deception by authority figures. When the general public believed that demons made them sick, exorcists made money selling holy water. Now we are bombarded with thousands of dietary solutions to our health problems, endorsed by genuine doctors and nutritionists—fat-melting miracle pills, detoxification smoothies, vitamin-rich goji berries—and we buy them, figuratively and literally. Frequently these solutions come packaged with a scapegoat. *Get rid of this one terrible substance and there will be no more cancer. No MSG, no headaches. Eliminate gluten, eliminate Alzheimer's. (And melt fat in the process!)* It's that simple: point an accusatory finger, tell the right story, and a new demon is born.

Like gluten today, MSG was once the scapegoat of choice. While debate about the dangers of MSG continued to rage in scientific journals, impatient doctors and eager advocates went public with premature conclusions. A mythic narrative quickly took shape, of virtuous researchers fighting against evil, baby-poisoning corporations. Media outlets played up the story's sensationalist allure, featuring hyperbolic headlines like this one from the *Chicago Tribune* in 1979: "Chinese food make you crazy? MSG is No. 1 Suspect."

Paranoia snowballed, and MSG metamorphosed from a potential allergen into a dietary supervillain. In 1988, Dr. George R. Schwartz, an emergency medicine specialist, published *In Bad Taste: The MSG Symptom Complex*, in which he connected MSG to the following ills: ADHD, AIDS, ALS, Alzheimer's, asthma, cancer, diarrhea, depression, gastroesophageal reflux, Huntington's, hyperactivity, hypertension, obesity, Parkinson's, and premenstrual syndrome.

Eight years later, neurosurgeon Russell L. Blaylock repackaged Schwartz's theories under the apocalyptic title *Excitotoxins: The Taste That Kills*. In his book, Blaylock provided a detailed "scientific" explanation of MSG's toxicity and addictiveness, and added autism to the list of ailments that it caused. Schwartz wrote the foreword, declaring *Excitotoxins* a "cutting-edge synthesis" by a "practicing, board-certified neurosurgeon with a deep understanding of the structure and function of the brain." He called for parents to stop poisoning their children, and predicted that Blaylock's book would be "seen as a landmark work" and "a marker of our time."

Schwartz's predictions did not come to pass. Instead, his license to treat patients was suspended in 2006 after authorities caught him illegally prescribing narcotics and amphetamines. (Schwartz still tweets sporadically from a Twitter account located in the "Mexican

Caribbean.") Blaylock is now a marginal figure in the anti-vaccine movement and the star of poorly produced YouTube videos like "Nutrition and the Illuminati Agenda." His most recent theory about our health problems singles out "chemtrails"—clouds of toxins spread secretly by government aircraft for undisclosed purposes.

Today these men look like obvious cranks. But in their time it was hard not to take them seriously. *In Bad Taste* and *Excitotoxins* overwhelmed readers with jargon and scientific citations, which, combined with the authors' medical pedigrees, created a compelling patina of authority. *60 Minutes* actually featured Schwartz in a 1991 segment on the dangers of MSG. When Jeff Nedelman, a spokesman for the Grocery Manufacturers Association, complained that Schwartz's appearance could lead to "unwarranted panic among consumers," he only reinforced the narrative of evil food companies fighting to keep consumers from the truth—just like tobacco companies had done when faced with damning evidence about cigarettes.

The case against MSG also drew strength from a common and convincing myth: *the products of technology and modernity are inherently dangerous*. Although ridiculous on its face—you wouldn't want to sip public drinking water from two hundred years ago—this myth has tremendous cultural currency. According to psychologist Keith Petrie at the University of Auckland, who specializes in how people perceive illness, fear of modernity routinely biases our judgments about medical care and dietary risk factors like MSG.

"Radio waves, chemicals—these things are invisible, and they are extremely powerful," Petrie explains to me. "That can be frightening. It makes you feel like you have no control of your health."

Schwartz and Blaylock expertly exploited their readers' fears of modernity. The ominous opening sentence of *Excitotoxins* uses the word "chemical" twice:

> What if someone were to tell you that a chemical added to food could cause brain damage in your children, and that this chemical could effect [sic] how your children's nervous systems formed during development so that in later years they may have learning or emotional difficulties?

Laypeople who struggled to understand Blaylock's technical case against MSG would have had no difficulty with his intuitive premise: modern substances—chemicals, additives, preservatives, vaccines, MSG—are inherently dangerous.

Belief in MSG's toxicity persists despite repeated debunkings. Scientists have confirmed and reconfirmed that the flavor enhancer, found in everything from sushi to Doritos, is no more suspicious than any other substance. In 2014, the American Chemical Society—the world's largest scientific organization—summarized the consensus yet again in a short video meant to reassure consumers that MSG is perfectly safe. Yet an online search turns up scores of popular articles that continue to regurgitate Schwartz's and Blaylock's unsubstantiated alarmism. One article for the Huffington Post calls MSG a "silent killer lurking in your kitchen cabinets." Another states that "chronic MSG ingestion by children may be one reason behind the nation's falling test scores." That's laughable, but not really surprising. For true believers, the myth will always be more sacred than the evidence.

For true believers, the myth will always be more sacred than the evidence.

If we are serious about the quest for good health, physical *and* mental, we cannot be slaves to fear and to our desire for easy answers. We must honestly admit our ignorance. We must recognize our capacity for self-deception. And when others—including medical and scientific professionals—refuse to do the same, we must learn to recognize their lies.

Sadly, the story of MSG is unexceptional in the world of nutrition science. Well-intentioned doctors constantly jump to unwarranted conclusions about food. Media outlets are always hungry for tales of crusaders fighting evil corporations. Supplement peddlers and diet gurus continue to exploit an irrational public. It would be nice if our current food fears were based on sound, settled science. But, as you are about to find out, nothing could be further from the truth. Most beliefs about gluten, fat, sugar, and salt have little basis in fact and everything to do with a powerful set of myths, superstitions, and lies, which, despite modern scientific progress, have remained unchanged for centuries.

This book is a call for change. Everyday foods don't have life-giving or death-dealing properties. Grocery stores aren't pharmacies. Your kitchen isn't stocked with silent killers, and the charlatans that make a living on false promises and uncertain science need to be revealed for what they really are. The time has come to slay our dietary demons, by exposing the falsehoods and liars that give them life.

CHAPTER ONE

Science Fiction Is Still Fiction

Monks Against the Grain

I am a scholar of religion. My job is to read sacred texts—myths, histories, commandments, prophecies—and then figure out what they meant and why they were persuasive. Although I specialize in classical Chinese thought, knowledge of other traditions informs my work. This is true for anyone who studies religion. If you are puzzling over the story of Noah's ark, it helps to examine similar flood myths, like the one in the Babylonian *Epic of Gilgamesh*, which comes complete with ark and animal rescue, or the one in the Hindu Mahabharata, where, in addition to rescuing animals, the hero saves the world's grains and seeds. The recurrence of this story, at different historical moments and with cultural variations, means that flood myths should be read as metaphors for divine punishment and cleansing, not as ancient weather reports. It also means that if a new myth surfaces about some forgotten North American flood, we probably shouldn't waste our time searching the Grand Canyon for the remains of an ark.

Religion and science are commonly understood to be separate explanatory systems, so my expertise may seem unrelated to nutrition. Modern debates about gluten, fat, sugar, and salt look scientific, not religious. They involve discussions of gut microbes and glucose, not gods and devils, and they draw evidence from peer-reviewed studies, not divine revelations. Again and again, the specialists I interviewed for this book asked how I ended up writing about a subject so different from what I typically study.

My answer was simple: I told them about the grain-free monks of ancient China. Like all diet gurus, these monks mocked the culinary culture of their time. They promised that a revolutionary diet could cure disease, quickly converting a substantial cult of followers. And, of course, they were wrong. The key to understanding and debunking fad diets, I suggested, wasn't science, but rather history. Once you see enough of the same archetypal myths and the same superstitions, new dietary claims start to look a lot like flood myths.

So what was going on with the grain-free monks? Two thousand years ago, the so-called five grains—two kinds of millet, hemp, rice, and beans—defined Chinese civilization. Early court historians used the adoption of agriculture and the cultivation of grains to distinguish civilized people from barbarians. Devotional poetry compared grains to the gods and praised them as the foundation of human life. To avoid the five grains was, quite literally, sacrilegious.

Yet a small minority of religious practitioners, the founders of Daoism, scandalized their contemporaries by referring to the five grains as "the scissors that cut off life." According to their radical teachings, conventional Chinese diets "rotted and befouled" your internal organs and led to disease and early death. Monks counseled seekers of long life to adopt a diet of plants gathered in the wild, supplemented with special minerals and exotic "elixirs," brewed according to proprietary alchemical formulas. The spectacular results of this strict regimen were documented in biographies of holy sages: perfect health, eternal youth, immortality, the ability to fly *and* teleport.

People in ancient China weren't stupid. Plenty of them doubted accounts of flying alchemists who never got sick. But despite basic logic and evidence to the contrary, the philosophy of the grain-free monks gained popularity. That's because then, as now, the appeal of dietary fads had to do with myths, not facts. In the case of the Daoists, grain prohibition represented rejection of modern culture and the promise of return to a mythic natural paradise. Suffering, disease, and death were ineradicable aspects of the present, so monks explained their dietary practices with an appealing fiction about a preagricultural paradise past.

When grains were the culinary symbol of Chinese civilization, Daoists argued that rejecting grains was the key to escaping modernity's ills. Later, when meat eating took on the symbolic importance once held by consuming grain, Daoist taboos shifted from the five grains to meat and blood. Rejection of the status quo—not science—determined the food prohibition du jour. But although the specific prohibition changed, the archetypal myth of a dietary route back to paradise remained constant, along with its false promises of eternal youth and perfect health.

The myth of paradise past is one of many irrational beliefs that recur across cultures and generations, influencing our attitude toward food. The history of dietary practices is full of superstition and magical thinking, from eating vegetarian because that's what Adam and Eve did in the Garden of Eden, to treating impotence with a tiger penis elixir. Once adopted, such practices become an important part of one's identity and therefore hard to question or give up. This is a version of what economists call the "sunk cost fallacy." When you embark on an elimination diet, you make a personal sacrifice along with a public declaration of your decision. Ending the diet means admitting your sacrifice was wasted and your decision was misguided—unpleasant considerations that favor continuing the diet, even if evidence comes out that it's unnecessary.

Rejecting a food—as the Daoist monks rejected grain—can also help define your membership in a superior group. We see this in the cross-cultural prevalence of food-based insults collected by anthropologists: "cannibals," "pork eaters," "sweet-potato eaters," "turtle eaters," "frog eaters," "locust eaters," "elephant eaters," "shit eaters," and so on. To begin eating a forbidden food means becoming a member of the group you once defined as inferior and unclean.

We may prefer to think that scientific progress has taken beliefs about food beyond myth and superstition. After all, the healthfulness of foods is now determined by scientific studies rather than holy texts, interpreted by people in lab coats instead of priestly robes. Reliable data on longevity have replaced anecdotes about long-lived monks. When secular authorities like the World Health Organization and the Food and Drug Administration dictate limits on fat, salt, and sugar, we assume their numbers reflect evidence-based knowledge.

In reality, scientifically established facts are only one of many factors influencing our dietary decisions. Modern American food discourse—including legal and scientific discourse—bristles with moral and religious vocabulary. Foods are "natural" or "unnatural," "good" or "bad." Bad foods may harm you, but they are "sinfully" delicious, "guilty" pleasures. Good foods, on the other hand, are "whole," "real," and "clean"—terms better suited to monastic manuals and philosophical treatises (what is *real* food, exactly?) than to scientific discussions.

These terms reflect our own idiosyncratic dietary faiths. Once, at a farmers' market, I asked a juice vendor whether her juice counted as "processed"—yet another vague, unscientific epithet that gets thrown around in discussions of food. After a moment of shock, she impressed upon me that processing fruit into juice doesn't result in processed food. Only corporations, she insisted, were capable of making processed food. Not only that, but it wasn't the processing that made something processed, so much as the presence of chemicals and additives.

Did the optional protein powder she offered count as a chemical additive, I pressed? A tan, gaunt customer interrupted us.

"It's easy," she said, staring at me intensely. "Processed food is evil."

Processed food is evil. Natural food is good. These are religious mantras, the condensed version of simplistic fairy tales that divide up foods, and the world, according to moralistic binaries. Genuine nutrition science, like all science, rejects oversimplification. "Natural" and "processed" are not scientific categories, and neither is good nor evil. These terms should be employed by monks and gurus, not doctors and scientists. Yet it is precisely such categories, largely unquestioned, that determine most people's supposedly scientific decisions about what and how to eat.

The Evolution of Food Myths

The unscientific basis of modern food beliefs features prominently in the work of Paul Rozin, a bearded, no-nonsense psychologist at the University of Pennsylvania. Rozin is best known for coining the phrase "the omnivore's dilemma"—which food writer Michael Pollan popularized as the title of his 2006 best seller—and he has written extensively about the influence of superstition on how we perceive what we eat.

"It's an immense problem," Rozin tells me, with the exasperated air of someone who must repeatedly explain a self-evident truth. "Love of

nature, it's like a religion. You can show that natural pesticides, whatever that means, are more dangerous than artificial ones, but it doesn't
matter. No one will believe you."

The mythic narrative of "unnatural" modernity and a "natural"
paradise past is persuasive as ever. Religious figures like Adam and Eve
are no longer plausible protagonists, so diet gurus replace them with
Paleolithic, preagricultural, hard-bodied ancestors who raced playfully
through the forest gathering berries and spearing wild boar, never once
worrying about diabetes or autism. The foods that belong to that culinary past are good. The products of modernity, by contrast—MSG,
grains, high-fructose corn syrup, genetically modified organisms, fast
food—these are the toxic fruits of sin, the tempting offerings of a fearsome deity known as Big Food.

Scientific rhetoric disguises the unscientific roots of modern food
fears. Saying we aren't *evolved* to eat gluten or processed sugar *sounds*
more factual than saying that God has forbidden them. But using the
language of science doesn't guarantee access to the insights of science.
In the case of unfounded dietary advice, it merely provides a new vocabulary with which to rewrite unscientific myths.

Although scientific training can inoculate against the power of
nutritional myths, by no means does it guarantee immunity. Science
is a way of understanding reality that relies on observation and experiment instead of moral judgments and intuition. But science is
practiced by humans, and humans can never fully bracket their irrational motivations. Researchers and doctors fear death and disease just
like everyone else. Many of them choose their careers out of the desire
to save people from needless suffering. So, when citizens and policy
makers clamor for solutions to public health crises, medical experts
can be tempted to overstate the extent of their knowledge and exagger-
ate the potential effects of dietary changes on health. The prospect of
healing the world with dietary laws has always been awfully appealing,

especially when those laws fit nicely with timeless myths or intuitive superstitions. The result is sloppy science: identify a suspicious substance, run a few studies that confirm what you set out to find, and presto, a new rule is born, sanctioned by reputable members of the scientific community. Don't eat too much salt. Don't eat too much fat. Don't eat sugar. Don't eat gluten.

Of course, anyone who pays attention to health news knows these rules can't be trusted. In 1984, an iconic *Time* magazine cover depicted a frowny face made of two eggs and a piece of bacon, under the tagline *Cholesterol—And Now the Bad News*. Thirty years later, the same magazine replaced the frowny face with a curl of butter, and changed the tagline to *Eat Butter*. "All red meat is risky, a study finds," reads a 2012 headline in the *Los Angeles Times*. But according to BBC Health News in 2013, fatty meat is "being . . . demonized" unfairly. And here's the *New York Times* on resveratrol, an organic compound found in red wine:

2011: "LONGER LIVES FOR OBESE MICE"

2012: "LIMITS TO RESVERATROL AS METABOLISM AID"

2013: "NEW OPTIMISM ON RESVERATROL"

2014: "WINE INGREDIENT MAY HAVE
FEW HEALTH BENEFITS"

Even so-called health foods offer no refuge. In 2014, *Vogue* magazine quotes Paleo guru Loren Cordain saying that quinoa "should be avoided." So what do we eat? Buttered bread and red wine or quinoa and lemon water? (Careful—lemon water eats away at your dental enamel.)

The problem here is that running a few studies doesn't "prove" or "conclusively show" *anything*. Good nutrition science depends on the long, slow accumulation of data over many, many studies, something scientists themselves know very well. They are highly skeptical—or should be—of single studies, in part thanks to a celebrated paper by Stanford professor John P. A. Ioannidis: "Why Most Published Research Findings Are False." Ioannidis's conclusion, helpfully summarized in the paper's title, explains what's really happening with the steady stream of scientific reversals on butter, wine, or whatever food appears in the latest headline: *In truth, there are no reversals occurring, because nothing was ever established in the first place.*

As you'll see in the following chapters, many researchers readily admit uncertainty about the health effects of gluten, fat, sugar, and salt. They are the honest ones. Enthusiastic gurus who speak confidently on the toxicity of sugar or the dangers of grains are exaggerating the state of the field—and exaggeration in science is nothing less than a lie. The problem is not with the scientific study of nutrition. The problem is people who misrepresent the strength of its findings.

Paradoxically, our faith in science makes it difficult to identify and dismiss lies about nutrition. Food seems simple to study. If we can put a man on the moon, transplant a heart, and manipulate DNA, then surely we can unpack the relationship between eating vegetables and living longer. There's no *obvious* difficulty in figuring out if wine decreases the risk of heart disease, or if red meat increases the risk of colon cancer. Just look at people who drink wine or eat red meat, and then compare them to those who don't. Easy, right?

In fact, there is probably no branch of medicine more difficult or complicated than nutrition science, a complexity that plays out in the endless controversies about what—and how much—we should eat. High-quality studies of dietary practices are incredibly hard to design. How do you make a placebo piece of steak for your control group? Studies on the effect of diet and lifestyle in large populations are no less difficult. They depend on recollection and self-reporting, notoriously unreliable data. And even if that data were accurate—well, just tweak an equation, exclude a set of data points, isolate a different factor, and suddenly vegetarianism goes from increasing longevity to decreasing bone density.

In dealing with these intractable problems of study design and analysis, nutrition scientists who study "ideal diets" have made surprisingly little progress since biblical days. According to the Hebrew Bible, the prophet Daniel and his fellow Israelites were once held captive by the king of Babylon. Loyal to Moses's dietary laws and afraid of defilement, Daniel requested what is almost certainly the first recorded trial of an elimination diet.

"Please test your servants for ten days," Daniel said to his guard. "Give us nothing but vegetables to eat and water to drink. Then compare our appearance with that of the young men who eat the royal food, and treat your servants in accordance with what you see."

The guard agreed. At the end of the ten days, Daniel and his friends "looked healthier and better nourished than any of the young men who ate the royal food." (It doesn't specify that their acne cleared up, but we can assume it did.)

Pre–twentieth century vegetarians cited Daniel as evidence of their diet's superiority. Nowadays they invoke people like Dr. Dean Ornish, a well-known advocate of veganism and meditation. Ornish has published studies in prestigious medical journals on how his regimen prevents cancer and heart disease. News outlets and TV shows tout his approach as a scientifically proven way to "reverse aging." They trust that his diet works, because unlike Daoist monks and biblical prophets, Ornish is a scientist and a doctor. But Ornish's studies, despite their author's pedigree, suffer from the same fundamental problems as Daniel's study: a lead investigator highly invested in the success of his experiment, the absence of a placebo control, and lack of replication by other researchers. In both cases it's impossible to distinguish between the actual power of vegetables and the effect of *believing* in the power of vegetables.

Time and time again, scientifically "proven" diets have proved false and foolish. At the turn of the twentieth century, health guru Horace Fletcher popularized his theory of mastication, which argued that good health depended on a low-protein diet, chewed hundreds of times before swallowing. Obese at age forty, "the Great Masticator" told a compelling story of his own dramatic weight loss by means of mastication. In addition to slimming down, he also became incredibly fit. To prove it, Fletcher submitted himself to tests of strength at Yale University, in which the fifty-year-old supposedly bested college athletes. And as if that wasn't enough, he mailed samples of his own stool to interested parties, the better to demonstrate the purity of his "digestive ash," which was "no more offensive than moist clay" and had "no more odor than a hot biscuit." *Nature will castigate those who don't masticate*, rhymed the eventual millionaire whose shit didn't stink.

This advice sounds ridiculous today, but among those who followed it were John D. Rockefeller, Franz Kafka, and pioneer of empirical psychology William James. You might think adherents of the latest dietary trend would learn from history and recognize that one day they could end up looking like disciples of the Great Masticator. But they don't. Studies keep appearing, headlines keep hyperbolizing, diet books top best-seller lists, and our faith that the newest fad will prove true remains unshaken.

The same is true of our belief in dietary demons like MSG and gluten. Population-wide studies of health and lifestyle have had some successes, most notably the discovery that cigarettes cause lung cancer. But the hunt for nutritional epidemiology's next tobacco has gone

remarkably poorly. In his book *Hyping Health Risks*, cancer epidemiologist Geoffrey Kabat puts it bluntly: The "low-hanging fruit" like
"smoking and lung cancer" have already been identified. With most
other risk factors, emphasizes Kabat, there is an "immense difficulty
[. . .] establishing credible linkages."

Eating in moderation has been the humdrum recommendation of
common sense for thousands of years, and to that sage dietary advice,
religion and science alike have added virtually nothing that stands up
to rigorous scrutiny. People who tell you otherwise are, at best, exaggerating evidence—and remember, in science, exaggeration is a flat-
out lie.

These lies aren't just misleading. They're bad for our culture and
our health. In hopes of escaping death and disease, we fawn over dietary evangelists with megawatt smiles and six-pack abs, each one
promising a different, revolutionary, "science-based" route to perfect
health. We embrace one food taboo after another, a habit that clinical psychologists condemn as conducive to disordered eating. Indeed,
in 2004, long before he was famous for telling the world to "eat food,
not too much, mostly plants," Michael Pollan railed against what he
called America's "national eating disorder." Citing the ridiculousness
of Horace Fletcher's mastication diet, he mused at our willingness to
embrace food fads and phobias.

"What is striking," Pollan wrote, "is just how little it takes to set
off one of these applecart-toppling nutritional swings in America; a
scientific study, a new government guideline, a lone crackpot with a
medical degree can alter this nation's diet overnight." He bemoaned
the growing trend of choosing food by the numbers—calories, carbs,
fats, RDAs—instead of choosing it with our senses. And he imagined
a future in which people judge food by its flavor, not its medicinal
value—where the ideal eater is a good home cook, not an expert in
paleoanthropology and nutrition science.

That future can't happen if we think our pantries are stocked with dietary demons and silent killers. And so I am hopeful that after I reveal the myths and superstitions behind fears of gluten, fat, sugar, and salt, you will be less afraid of these vilified foods—and food in general.

Without fear, not only will eating be more pleasurable, it may also be more healthful. As Paul Rozin likes to remind people, "Worrying about food is not good for you." He suggests that the cause of expanding waistlines and exploding hearts in America isn't necessarily what we eat but *how* we eat—anxiously, obsessed with nutrition, counting calories, scanning food labels, eliminating foods and then bingeing on them. We are vigilant over what goes into our mouths, at the cost of vigilance over what goes into our minds, shunning junk food while bingeing on bad science.

Fiction, not food, is the real demon. Like the hucksters of our recent past and the grain-free monks of ancient China, the latest set of gurus and government guidelines pollutes our culture with new versions of the same timeless falsehoods. Gluten belongs to the fallen present, not paradise past. If you eat fat, you will become fat. Processed sugar is "unnatural." Big Food murders infants with high-sodium baby food. These falsehoods produce paralyzing anxiety about food and a constant stream of contradictory claims about what we should eat, which in turn erodes public faith in the enterprise of science itself.

Enough is enough. In order to heal our culture we must counteract the standard American diet of food myths with healthy helpings of history and skepticism. These ingredients may taste unusual at first, but don't worry—it won't be long before you feel like a brand-new person, capable of laughing at the latest nutrition nonsense and eating your dinner in peace.

CHAPTER TWO

The Gluten Lie

The Gluten Liars

Kristin Voorhees's earliest memories are of sitting on the toilet, doubled over in pain, holding her parents' hands. Her childhood was a litany of health woes: colic as an infant, recurring strep throat, constant stomach pain, irritable bowel syndrome, acid reflux. In sixth grade she developed a severe rash on her legs, and in high school her thyroid swelled up. A parade of doctors prescribed antibiotics for the strep, esomeprazole for the acid reflux, and administered a battery of tests to figure out what was wrong. They failed.

"I was told, 'You have IBS.' 'You have lactose intolerance,'" Kristin recounts to me. "One of the gastroenterologists reading a lab report told me I was crazy. I remember it as clear as day, Thanksgiving of my senior year, and he told me I was crazy, I was nuts, and I should just get over it."

During her time at James Madison University, Kristin saw a total of seven different physicians, constantly traveling home to New Jersey from Virginia in hopes that someone would be able to stop the pain and bloating and give her back her life. Finally, just after graduation, she was awakened by a phone call. It was the physician from the latest lab.

"He said, 'We're pretty sure you have something called celiac disease,'" Kristin recalls. "Then he said, 'Go on the Internet and look it up.' No help, no instructions, nothing. I decided to go shopping, and I remember crying in the dressing room, wanting to stop for food and not knowing what to do."

Kristin is one of many genetically predisposed individuals for whom gluten and related proteins cause a dangerous autoimmune reaction. The symptoms range widely, from acute gastrointestinal pain and skin rashes to increased risk for certain cancers, infertility, and neurological disorders. Research suggests that almost one in a hundred Americans—3 million—may be affected by celiac disease (CD). Of these, only 17 percent are diagnosed, which means 2.5 million Americans might be living with undiagnosed CD—a huge number that the National Foundation for Celiac Awareness is working tirelessly to shrink. (Kristin is currently the NFCA's director of health-care initiatives.)

On top of that, a slightly larger number of Americans who don't have CD may experience symptoms after ingesting gluten, usually joint pain, fatigue, "foggy mind," or numbness of their extremities. This is referred to as non-celiac gluten sensitivity (NCGS), a condition that remains a matter of considerable debate. (We'll return to NCGS in a moment.)

Yet CD and NCGS alone don't explain the astonishing prevalence of anti-gluten sentiment. According to industry analysts, almost one-third of Americans want to cut down on gluten or avoid it entirely. That means steering clear of all foods made with wheat and related grains, which requires serious sacrifice. The Celiac Disease Foundation provides a partial list of common offenders: raviolis, dumplings, couscous, gnocchi, ramen, udon, soba noodles, croissants, pita, naan, bagels, corn bread, muffins, doughnuts, pretzels, Goldfish, graham crackers, cakes, cookies, pies, brownies, pancakes, waffles, French toast, crepes, croutons, soy sauce, cream sauces with roux, beer.

In addition, those who eat gluten-free have to cultivate wariness and endless vigilance: potato chips, tortilla chips, salad dressings, french fries, meat substitutes, cheesecake, and virtually any restaurant dish often conceal gluten. (Catholic sufferers need to check on their communion wafers.)

Since people desperately miss these culinary delights, the global market for gluten-free alternatives has grown to around $4 billion, and is projected to reach nearly $7 billion by 2019. Many Walmarts now dedicate precious floor space to gluten-free shopping. You can even buy various kinds of gluten-free dog food, though veterinary scientists have only identified gluten sensitivity in Irish setters. And all this gluten-free living comes at a premium. According to a 2008 study of two large-chain general grocery stores, gluten-free products were, on average, 242 percent more expensive than their regular counterparts.

Gluten-free products were, on average, 242 percent more expensive than their regular counterparts.

So why are more than 80 million Americans without CD or NCGS eager to embrace such a difficult and costly dietary regimen? The very latest surge of interest can be traced to the massive influence of Dr. William Davis and Dr. David Perlmutter, the authors of the blockbuster best sellers *Wheat Belly* and *Grain Brain*, respectively. According to Davis and Perlmutter, avoiding gluten isn't just for people with CD or NCGS. Their shocking theories assert that gluten-containing grains cause or exacerbate a laundry list of ailments: ADHD, Alzheimer's, arthritis, autism, cancer, heart disease, obesity, schizophrenia, and pretty much anything else you've ever worried about. As Davis puts it in a characteristic sentence from *Wheat Belly*: "Increased estrogen, breast cancer, man boobs . . . all from the bag of bagels shared at the office."

Wheat Belly and *Grain Brain* make the case that mainstream doctors and the USDA, long in the pocket of the food industry, have been complicit in the greatest health scandal since tobacco. Bread, the staff of life, is really the staff of *death*. The science, they say, is clear: every time you drink a beer or eat a flour tortilla you are poisoning yourself with a toxin more addictive and dangerous than cocaine. Sporting an impressive set of citations and filled with technical terms like *leptin* and *gliadin*, the books ooze scientific integrity like your wheat belly oozes over your belt. No wonder so many Americans are interested in cutting down on gluten.

We should know better. For one, the recent demonization of gluten looks suspiciously like the misguided demonization of MSG. Two doctors become instant media darlings, despite neither being a leader in his field, much less an expert in nutrition science (Davis is a cardiologist, Perlmutter is a neurologist). In TV and radio interviews, no mention is made of Perlmutter's dubious early work—pop-science books packed with alarmism and outrageous promises. "Is your cell phone frying your brain?" he asks in *The Better Brain Book* (2005). (Almost certainly, and so is your clock radio. Watch out!) "Raise IQ by up to 30 points and turn on your child's smart genes," guarantees the subtitle of *Raise a Smarter Child by Kindergarten* (2008). Tell us about gluten, Doctor! Will eliminating it help boost my child's IQ?

Then there are the websites. Perlmutter's dubs him "an empowering neurologist," and visitors can choose from a selection of Perlmutter-branded nutritional supplements like Empowering Brain Formula ($73.95). Not to be outdone, William Davis's website advertises him as a "health crusader." There, visitors can browse recipes, watch a clip of Davis on *The Dr. Oz Show*, and subscribe to his monthly wellness community called "Cureality" for $9.95/month. The marketplace section of Cureality.com is obviously a work in progress, but members can still score discounts on fish oil and home blood tests.

Make no mistake: despite their credentials, these men are sensationalists, not scientists. Citations and jargon notwithstanding, their books are filled with slick, manipulative, unscientific hyperbole, designed to scare the crap out of you and make their authors money. What's shocking isn't their theories—it's that so many people take them seriously.

Knowing about the power of myth helps explain readers' gullibility. The first sentences of Davis's and Perlmutter's introductions are eerily similar, as if taken from some master manual of pseudoscientific mythmaking. Each reinforces the lie that the past was better—safer, healthier—than the present:

> *Wheat Belly*: "Flip through your parents' or grandparents' family albums and you're likely to be struck by how *thin* everyone looks."

> *Grain Brain*: "If you could ask your grandparents or great-grandparents what people died from when they were growing up, you'd likely hear the words 'old age.'"

Of course, if you walk through a graveyard, you'll be struck by the tiny tombstones from your great-grandparents' generation, when infants and children died far more frequently than today. If you flip through old photo albums, you'll eventually come across victims of polio lying in iron lungs—a problem we no longer face thanks to vaccines. And you probably don't give a second thought to typhoid fever, dysentery, and cholera, because in 1908 health officials began purifying our drinking water with a scary chemical called chlorine.

Davis and Perlmutter egregiously misrepresent the reality of the past—and, as we are about to see, they are no better on the present. At best *Wheat Belly* and *Grain Brain* are collections of unfounded speculations, cherry-picked data, and overconfident hypotheses. At worst they are tantamount to medical malpractice, snake oil in literary form that should earn the authors the censure of their professional peers. Instead, they're earning millions of dollars and a loyal following of converts who believe in their saviors with the intensity of religious zealots. As one commenter writes breathlessly on Perlmutter's website: "Your book is like my bible right now. It has literally changed my life. I can't thank you enough."

It's about time these false prophets get exposed for what they really are, so people can ignore them. Only then will we understand the truth about gluten and be free to make dietary decisions based on sound science.

What Real Experts Say About Gluten

I know that by criticizing Perlmutter and Davis I risk committing sacrilege. Thousands of people feel they owe their lives to these men. You, my reader, might be among them. Maybe you did "lose the wheat" and "lose the weight"—or discovered that forgoing bread and pasta left you feeling healthier and happier than ever before. Maybe you haven't read these books, but found tremendous relief by going gluten-free, even though doctors tested you for CD and the test came back negative. You may be sick of being told by experts that the problems in your gut are really "in your head." You might be certain that, time and time again, your stomach has revolted against the hidden gluten in foods like soy sauce when you had no idea it was there.

If so, please hear me out. I'm not saying you are crazy or denying your health struggles. Your diarrhea was not "in your head." And I am not here to declare that gluten sensitivity doesn't exist. I don't believe the reports, widely circulated on social media, that some study proved "non-celiac gluten sensitivity is fake." In fact, I have spoken extensively with Dr. Peter Gibson, coauthor of the study responsible for those reports, who confirmed his work proves no such thing.

Yet Gibson and countless experts on CD and gluten roundly *reject* the theses of Davis and Perlmutter. Gastroenterologists are nearly unanimous in their reluctance to recommend "trying out" a gluten-free diet. Dr. Stefano Guandalini, medical director of the University of Chicago Celiac Disease Center, said flatly in 2013 that "it is not a healthier diet for those who don't need it." Millions who give up bread and hunt for gluten-free toothpaste, he opined, "are following a fad, essentially."

Shouldn't we trust him—an expert dedicated to the treatment of celiac disease—at least as much as we trust a self-proclaimed "health crusader" and a neurologist who makes his money peddling Empowering Brain Formula?

And it's not just Guandalini who urges caution when it comes to going gluten-free. Physicians who actually focus on their patients' well-being don't want them to waste energy and money on a needless elimination diet. In a 2013 state-of-the-field collection of essays, *A Clinical Guide to Gluten-Related Disorders*, the authors recommend confirming a diagnosis of CD before "embarking on treatment," which can be "burdensome to follow and adds significantly to the cost of living." The preface to *A Clinical Guide* describes the theory that gluten contributes to Alzheimer's and schizophrenia—*grain brain!*—as "particularly controversial." It also emphasizes that many "fantasies" are associated with non-celiac gluten sensitivity, and urges a cautious, science-based approach to the condition.

These experts are not pawns of Big Food or naive physicians hamstrung by conventional thinking. (Nor do they run websites that hawk dietary supplements and gluten-free cookbooks.) *A Clinical Guide* was edited by gastroenterologist Dr. Alessio Fasano, director of the Mucosal Immunology and Biology Research Center and the Center for Celiac Research and Treatment at Massachusetts General Hospital. Fasano is among the world's most influential CD researchers and an outspoken advocate for awareness of non-celiac gluten sensitivity. Many citations at the back of *Wheat Belly* and *Grain Brain* refer to studies conducted by him.

If anything, *A Clinical Guide* overstates the evidence for NCGS. The book includes a full section devoted to it, in which Dr. Carlo Catassi and Dr. Anna Sapone write that "the positive effect of a gluten withdrawal in [NCGS] patients cannot be entirely explained by a placebo effect." To justify their conclusion, they cite a double-blind, randomized, placebo-controlled study—the "gold standard" of dietary studies—which found that "irritable bowel–like symptoms of gluten sensitivity were more frequent in the gluten-treated group (68 percent) than in the subjects on placebo (40 percent)." Conducted at Australia's Monash University, the study received considerable attention. Many people, including Catassi and Sapone, took it to confirm that non-celiac gluten sensitivity is, in at least some cases, a physiological condition. Science had shown that just because you don't have CD doesn't mean your gluten sensitivity is all in your head.

But after *A Clinical Guide* had gone to print, the same researchers at Monash conducted another study that came to a remarkably different conclusion. Using an even more rigorous trial design, they found there were "no effects of gluten in patients with self-reported non-celiac gluten sensitivity." The authors hypothesized that gluten sensitivity was actually being confused with sensitivity to special carbohydrates known as FODMAPs (short for fermentable oligo-, di-, mono-saccharides and polyols). While FODMAPs are found in grains such as wheat, rye, and barley, they also occur in a wide variety of "gluten-free" or "healthy" foods like broccoli, garlic, onions, apples, and avocados. In other words: those who think they have NCGS may be reacting to what's inside their sandwiches as much as the bread itself.

Both of the Monash studies were coauthored by Peter Gibson, director of gastroenterology at the Alfred Hospital and Monash University, who has been trying to cut through the media hyperbole and clarify what the back-and-forth really means.

"People said the researchers in Australia have changed their minds," Gibson complains to me. "They don't understand what science is. We didn't change our minds. We just produced more data. You don't come into research as an evangelist—otherwise you start to misinterpret your own data. We're just looking for the truth, and the truth right now is that we've just scratched the surface."

Gibson, who helped develop the low-FODMAP diet, was understandably excited by the results of the second study, which suggested that some people who go gluten-free might be better off on a low-FODMAP diet. But during our conversation he repeated, emphatically, that *nothing had been proved*, and he had little patience for books like *Grain Brain* and *Wheat Belly*, which he felt distorted the evidence and reflected poorly on a scientific community genuinely invested in discovery, not sensationalism.

"These books, they're usually convincingly written," Gibson says. "But they use science in an inappropriate way—we just call it pseudoscience—saying 'this' causes 'that' because 'this' has been observed. The link can be very tenuous, but it makes for a great story. Most of it is just anecdotes and big ideas."

Getting at the Truth

According to scientists like Gibson who are at the forefront of gluten research, the conclusions in *Wheat Belly* and *Grain Brain* are premature and irresponsible. They are convincing not because of their basis in sound science, but rather because they reinforce powerful myths and promise simple dietary solutions to a variety of health problems.

It is crucial to debunk these books and the empire they have spawned—not just for the sake of setting the scientific record straight, but because alarmist rhetoric can make people physically and mentally ill. A significant minority benefits from a gluten-free diet. But for everyone else, exaggerating the danger posed by gluten isn't merely speculation—it is actively harmful. Ironically, anxiety about what you eat can produce precisely the same symptoms linked to gluten sensitivity. Demonizing food can contribute to the development of eating disorders. And, perhaps most worryingly, the logic of charlatans who embrace untested "revolutionary truths" over "conventional wisdom" licenses dangerous behavior like refusing to vaccinate children. Why trust establishment stooges, right? They're the same ones who told us to eat toxic, gluten-containing foods so Big Pharma could keep pumping us full of medicine, insulin, and vaccines.

Anxiety about what you eat can produce precisely the same symptoms linked to gluten sensitivity.

No one wants to support merchants of fear and false hope. We have the right to know what's actually going on with our bodies, and we shouldn't have to abandon our favorite foods if there's nothing wrong with them. There's no reason to see hamburger buns as silent killers, especially if—as I will discuss later in this chapter—food anxiety is a possible health threat. In what follows, I hope to help you recognize lies about gluten—the lies you may tell yourself, and the lies you are told by friends, family, the media, and even unscrupulous medical professionals.

Because this is history, not fiction, you won't read about a paradise past in which lithe Paleolithic humans lived free from Alzheimer's and irritable bowel syndrome, eating only what nature provided. There is no USDA or FDA conspiracy. There are no miracle cures and no easy answers. There is only the truth: about how we came to fear gluten, and why, for the majority of us, that fear has no foundation in fact.

I wish I could offer up a single nutritional scapegoat to blame for conditions like autism and Alzheimer's, cancer and arthritis. *"Why do I and my loved ones suffer and die?"* is the most urgent question one can ask, and simple dietary answers—MSG or gluten or whatever comes next—give us comfort. Unfortunately, those simple answers are not real solutions. The subtitle of *Grain Brain* is "the surprising truth about wheat, carbs, and sugar—your brain's silent killers." But the actual truth is that *Grain Brain* is a lie, and our best science just doesn't know what causes many of our most serious afflictions.

That doesn't mean there's no hope. Medical knowledge is constantly advancing, thanks to tireless research by scientists genuinely concerned with discovering the truth. In December 2013, a drug called sofosbuvir was approved to treat hepatitis C. The treatment has a cure rate of over 90 percent, a life-changing breakthrough for the 3.2 million Americans with the disease. And in September 2014, the son of actor Christopher Reeve announced a huge advance in the treatment of spinal injury called epidural stimulation. Four young men, told they would never move again below their neck or chest, regained the ability to stand and move their hips, legs, and toes. They also regained bowel control, bladder control, and sexual function.

As I write these words, Reeve's foundation is busy raising $15 million to test the treatment on thirty-six more paralyzed men and women. If everyone who bought a copy of *Wheat Belly* had donated their money instead, the study would be funded. And studying gluten-free diets costs far less—the same amount would have funded at least a hundred studies at Monash University, the Center for Celiac Research and Treatment, or James Cook University, where researchers recently found that infecting celiac patients with hookworm dramatically increased their ability to tolerate gluten.

I'm confident that one day we will know much more about NCGS, and we may even be able to effectively treat celiac disease. I'm also confident we will make great strides treating Alzheimer's, autism, cancer, and other intractable medical conditions. But in the meantime, there's no need for people to give up their grains. Trust the researchers, not the "empowering health crusaders." Going gluten-free isn't going to shrink your man boobs or heal your child's autism. And if you don't trust the researchers, trust the lessons of history. You see, it turns out this isn't the first time a treatment meant for CD was touted as an unsubstantiated panacea and weight-loss miracle.

That honor, weirdly, belongs to bananas.

A Brief History of Celiac Disease

In 1887, Dr. Samuel Gee gave the first comprehensive description of what he called the "coeliac affection" at the Hospital for Sick Children in London. Coeliac, or celiac as it is now commonly spelled, means "sickness of the belly" in Greek. Gee observed that certain people suffered from a terrible wasting disease marked by the production of "whitish stinking stool." The afflicted, mostly children, suffered horribly: muscle aches, weakness, wild swings in appetite, stunted growth. "The course of the disease is always slow," wrote Gee. "Whether the patient live or die, he lingers ill for months and years."

As to what caused the condition, Gee could only speculate. Nevertheless, he concluded that "if the patient can be cured at all, it must be by means of diet." His own prescription prohibited cows' milk, fruits, and vegetables, preferring "asses' milk," "bread cut thin and well toasted on both sides," and even "a quart of the best Dutch mussels daily." (This last was a formula with which Gee had success on one occasion—but he was never able to repeat it.)

After Gee, the most influential account of CD was the 1908 book *On Infantilism from Chronic Intestinal Infection*, written by Christian

Herter, a physician and professor at Columbia University. But despite the work of these two pioneers, the medical community remained mystified by what became known as "Gee-Herter disease." Hypothesized causes ranged from viral and bacterial infection to malfunction of the liver or pancreas. Due to the presence of excess fat in the feces of celiac sufferers, a low-fat diet was thought to be helpful, and a 1939 British review of seventy-three cases pronounced a "low-fat diet with added vitamins" the best method of treatment.

The mystery ended with Dutch physician Willem Dicke. The medical director of Juliana Children's Hospital in The Hague, Dicke first became interested in CD after attending a meeting of pediatricians in 1932. There, a colleague described relapses of diarrhea in a celiac patient who had consumed bread. Dicke began experimenting with wheat-free diets, carefully documenting reactions to individual foods in his patients. In 1941, he published a report about his successes. "I give a simple diet," wrote Dicke, " . . . [that] should not contain any bread or rusks. A hot meal twice a day is also well tolerated. The third meal can be sweet or sour porridge (without any wheat flour)."

Linking wheat flour to CD was a revolutionary thesis, and the end of World War II provided additional evidence to confirm it. Due to a German embargo and a severe winter, the western Netherlands plunged into famine at the end of 1944, a period known as the *Hongerwinter* (hunger winter). Children everywhere were starving, but, paradoxically, celiac patients appeared to be improving. In 1945, the hunger winter ended with bread drops over Holland. A blessing to most of the starving children, the bread produced relapses in celiac patients, who until that time had no access to any food made with wheat flour.

Following World War II, Dicke and colleagues performed experiments that identified gluten as the cause of malabsorption in celiacs. This, not excess fat in the diet, was responsible for the fat typically found in the feces of patients. Then, in 1956, British physician Margot

Shiner pioneered the use of intestinal biopsy capsules, which led to conclusive evidence that gluten altered the intestinal mucosa in celiac patients. Before long, the international medical community quickly adopted gluten-free diets to treat celiac disease.

Well, most of the international community. In America, grave doubts persisted about Dicke's approach, due to the continuing influence of a prominent pediatrician and CD researcher named Sidney V. Haas. Now relegated to footnotes, Haas had pioneered a treatment for CD known as "the banana diet," which he first detailed in a 1924 article for the *American Journal of Diseases of Children*. Haas's theories about bananas are now obsolete, but the story of his diet is prophetic.

Gluten-free Is . . . Bananas?

At the turn of the twentieth century, the United Fruit Company mounted an aggressive advertising campaign to complement its increased capacity to grow and import bananas. With the fruit no longer an exotic luxury, United Fruit took advantage of testimonials by doctors and nutritionists to reimagine bananas as a superfood—the acai or goji berries of the early twentieth century. A 1917 industry publication, *Food Value of the Banana*, included a glowing endorsement from the *Journal of the American Medical Association*: "This fruit is sealed by nature in practically germ-free and germ-proof packages." Numerous dietitians testified to their curative powers. It was only logical for Haas to try them with celiac patients, and he started a few of them on a strict diet of bananas and milk, supplemented with broth, gelatin, and a little meat.

The results were astonishing. Of ten children treated, eight experienced dramatic symptom remission and dramatically increased height and weight. (According to Haas, the two that died failed to comply with his regimen.) Haas's 1924 article described these results in hyperbolic terms accompanied by impressively detailed charts, nutritional breakdowns of the diet, and before-and-after photographs of strikingly transformed children.

In all likelihood, Haas's young patients really did experience miraculous transformations, since they were no longer eating gluten. But Haas didn't know about gluten's role in celiac, so he came up with an unsubstantiated theory that bananas contain a special enzyme "capable of hydrolyzing" starch and "of converting cane sugar to invert sugar." This enzyme, not the absence of gluten, was thought to be the primary driver of his children's recovery.

Validated by Haas's success treating children with CD, bananas and the banana diet became increasingly popular. At Johns Hopkins, Dr. George Harrop tried a simplified version of the banana diet on diabetics and found that while their diabetes remained unresolved, they lost a lot of weight. Harrop published his results in 1934. The public, predictably, went bananas.

Overnight, the "bananas and skim milk" diet became a weight-loss craze. Like many low-carb, gluten-free enthusiasts today, fans of the banana diet extolled its ability to keep them satiated. One Milwaukee newspaper reported that women following it "do not go hungry" and "never have that pinched, ravenous feeling." Incredibly, it is still recommended on some mainstream health websites. Livestrong.com concludes that the diet "will result in dramatic weight loss, but may also make you irritable," and recommends dieters "drink plenty of water as bananas can be constipating."

Part of the diet's allure was due to the banana's existing status as a superfood. After Haas had developed the banana diet, United Fruit parlayed the fruit's ability to fight CD into more general claims about its healthfulness. One emeritus Harvard Medical School professor remarked in 1932 that the medical literature concerning the banana diet read less like science and more "like advertisements of the United Fruit Company." But the opinion of the medical community was drowned out by enthusiastic newspaper headlines like "Bananas Help Ill Child" (in a 1932 edition of the *New York Times*). Such reports confirmed the amazing powers of bananas to an uncritical public, who happily generalized the therapeutic properties of bananas to themselves.

World War II brought further opportunities for banana propaganda. American fruit ships were converted into military carriers, the railroad system was overwhelmed, and bananas became scarce. *Newsweek* and the *New York Times* described the odyssey of mothers searching neighborhoods for hours, desperate for bananas to feed their celiac-stricken infants. Soon after, a letter written by Haas appeared in the *Times*, assuring everyone that United Fruit was "doing all that is possible to meet the situation." Since CD was thought to be very rare at the time, the United Fruit Company made sure to complement stories about the treatment of celiac with more general claims about the healthfulness of bananas, continually invoking nutrient density and high concentrations of calories and vitamins.

Their strategy worked. The mythic superiority of bananas, based in part on their ability to treat CD, had incredible staying power. Working in the early 1960s, pediatrician William Brady wrote newspaper articles and a book advising mothers to "begin feeding the baby banana at the age of four or five weeks instead of four or five months," a program sure to make "puny, sickly, badly nourished infants thrive." Anecdotes of bananas' benefits abounded. "A Minnesota mother," gushed Brady, "started her three babies on banana when they were about two weeks old." The result? "None of the babies ever had a 'colic,' a laxative, an enema, or a suppository, and at the age of five or six weeks they all slept through the night." Bananas had gone from a prescription for celiac to a miracle that prevented colic and made babies sleep through the night.

Disappointingly for United Fruit, Dicke's research in the Netherlands proved that bananas had no special powers. The benefits of Haas's

treatment were due to the accidental prohibition of gluten. Haas, understandably, didn't want to give up his status as a trailblazing savior,
and resisted this development to the bitter end. He claimed that gluten-
free diets were prone to failure. He argued that they treated symptoms
instead of the underlying cause—an oft-used mantra in the condemnation of "conventional" medicine. Only the banana diet, said Haas,
could achieve a "cure which is permanent without relapse."

As celiac patients now know, he
was wrong. Currently celiac disease
is incurable. The only known treatment is abstaining from gluten. Bananas, sadly, are just bananas. That
much we've learned. What we haven't
learned, apparently, is the ability to be
skeptical. Here's what happened with

> **Currently celiac
> disease is incurable.
> The only known
> treatment is abstaining
> from gluten.**

the banana diet: A treatment originally meant for celiac patients turned
into a weight-loss fad. People ended up believing that if something can
help with CD, it can also help with all sorts of unrelated conditions.

Sound familiar?

From Treating Celiac Disease to Treating Everything

Less attached to the banana diet than its inventor, the medical community left Haas behind and endorsed going gluten-free as the proper
treatment for celiac disease. Strangely, the consequences for celiac sufferers in America were disastrous. United Fruit stopped invoking CD
in its ads, and people forgot about the disease almost entirely. Americans authored only 1 percent of research articles on CD between 1966
and 1995. There were no mentions of the disease in newspapers or
magazines between 1964 (the occasion of Sidney Haas's obituary) and
1980. As a result, millions of Americans went undiagnosed. Patients
had their CD mistaken for ulcerative colitis, Crohn's disease, irritable

bowel syndrome, and other food intolerances, which often led to serious complications and unnecessary surgeries.

One of those patients was a four-year-old named Judy, the daughter of Elaine Gottschall, a New Jersey housewife. In 1955, Judy began suffering from severe chronic intestinal distress and bleeding, which specialists diagnosed as incurable ulcerative colitis. Gottschall watched, powerless, as her daughter developed neurological problems and suffered stunted growth. Three years after the initial diagnosis, when steroid treatment and other pharmaceuticals proved ineffective, doctors told Gottschall the only solution was to surgically remove Judy's colon and equip her with a colostomy bag. No one ever thought to diagnose Judy with CD. She never tried going gluten-free.

Desperate for an alternative, Gottschall found her way to a ninety-two-year-old physician practicing in New York City: Sidney V. Haas. Immediately upon seeing Judy, Haas prescribed his banana diet. Within ten days Judy began to bounce back. Two years later she was symptom-free.

Haas's diet saved Gottschall's daughter from surgery and possibly death. It is therefore no surprise that Gottschall became an ardent defender of Haas's theories. Justifiably frustrated by the medical establishment that had repeatedly failed her, Gottschall was quick to blame widespread acceptance of Dicke's gluten-free diet on character flaws, not scientific consensus. She accused doctors of being attracted to Dicke's approach because of intellectual laziness, and rejected the idea that celiac disease should be treated by going gluten-free.

In 1968, four years after Haas's death, Gottschall went back to school at the urging of her husband, earning a bachelor's degree in biology and a master's degree in nutritional biochemistry and cellular biology. Drawing on her own research, Gottschall eventually wrote two books, *Food and the Gut Reaction*, published in 1992, and then her best seller, *Breaking the Vicious Cycle*, published in 1994. Inspired by Haas,

Breaking the Vicious Cycle argues that only the "specific carbohydrate diet"—a highly restrictive regimen that eliminates most starches, including potatoes and rice—can truly "cure" CD, as well as a variety of other disorders, the cause and treatment of which continue to bedevil most "conventional" doctors: Crohn's, ulcerative colitis, inflammatory bowel disease, irritable bowel syndrome, non-specific chronic diarrhea, obesity, and brain function disorders like epilepsy. The most recent edition of *Breaking the Vicious Cycle* adds a chapter on autism, claiming in no uncertain terms that the specific carbohydrate diet "has been effective in the treatment of autism."

The appeal of Gottschall's book is easy to understand, since it invokes the classic myths that characterize bad nutrition science:

> The Specific Carbohydrate Diet is biologically correct because it is species appropriate. The allowed foods are mainly those that early man ate before agriculture began. The diet we evolved to eat over millions of years was predominantly one of meat, fish, eggs, vegetables, nuts, low-sugar fruits. [. . .] In the last hundred years the increase in complex sugars and chemical additives in the diet has led to a huge increase in health problems ranging from severe bowel disorders to obesity and brain function disorders. We have not adapted to eat this modern diet as there has not been enough time for natural selection to operate.

Here, laid out succinctly, is the myth of paradise past that underlies every single blockbuster diet of the last decade, from the Paleo diet, which literally takes its name from the imperative to "eat like early man," to the wheat- and grain-elimination diets advocated by Davis and Perlmutter. Modernity is dangerous and unnatural, and the solution to numerous, fearsome ailments lies in returning to the lifestyle of paradise past. It is this myth that rationalizes the move from a diet meant for celiac disease to a dietary panacea—and people just eat it up.

Indeed, the same myth powers the first book-length argument against eating gluten-containing grains. In 2002, Dr. James Braly and Ron Hoggan published *Dangerous Grains*—unmentioned in *Grain Brain* and *Wheat Belly*—which contains the seeds of every modern anti-gluten argument. The first chapter is titled "Grains and People: An Evolutionary Mismatch." Another chapter, "Brain Disorders and Gluten," outlines what Perlmutter would later turn into an entire book. The authors bring up "opioid-peptides" that "look and act just like . . . morphine"—subsequently singled out by William Davis in *Wheat Belly* for the supposed addictiveness of modern "Frankenwheat."

In light of these "scientific facts," Hoggan and Braly assert that a large portion of the population, if not everyone, would benefit from a gluten-free diet. It's all right there—the same line of thinking, the same evidence. So who were these revolutionary thinkers that pre-empted Davis and Perlmutter by a decade? Were they well-established researchers with decades of experience?

Though he coauthored a groundbreaking treatise on *the* health threat of our time, I could not locate Dr. Braly at any research insti-tution. (His September 2014 LinkedIn profile lists him as director of the now-defunct Stem Cell Research Center of North America—once located in Tijuana, Mexico.)

But I was able to track down Braly's coauthor, Ron Hoggan, who still writes online columns and speaks at CD community events.

"I essentially wrote the book, and Dr. Braly was just going to be the promotional guy," Hoggan tells me. "I would do the writing, send it off to Dr. Braly, and he would go through it. He added a lot of adjectives in his editing."

Like Gottschall, Hoggan's motivations for writing the book were intensely personal. Labeled "emotional, picky, fussy, attention-seeking, and a hypochondriac," he moved from one misdiagnosis to the next, all the while suffering from chronic back and leg pain, hand tremors, and heartburn. At long last, in 1994, Hoggan was diagnosed with celiac disease, and after he adopted a gluten-free diet, his symptoms vanished.

Hoggan knew his brother, Jack, suffered from symptoms related to CD, and encouraged him to get tested. Jack refused to listen (a common reaction in families where one member is diagnosed with celiac). Eventually Hoggan's brother died of non-Hodgkin's lymphoma, a form of cancer for which the relative risk is four times higher in untreated CD sufferers than in the general population.

Devastated by his brother's death, Hoggan devoted his life to publicizing the risks associated with CD and grain consumption. Following the same course as Elaine Gottschall, he returned to school and earned a master's degree, and he, too, developed a distrust of the medical establishment. This distrust worsened when a pathologist refused to diagnose his daughter with celiac disease, leading to "months of depression, lethargy, and abdominal pain," before a second opinion confirmed her condition. *Dangerous Grains* was Hoggan's way of taking matters into his own hands, and redeeming the suffering and death of his family members.

It is extremely likely that others have gone through an experience similar to Hoggan's. Research is beginning to demonstrate a high prevalence of undiagnosed CD in sufferers of fibromyalgia, irritable bowel syndrome, diabetes, atopic eczema, and other related conditions. If estimates of celiac prevalence are accurate, and only 17 percent of sufferers are diagnosed, that means a large number of individuals whose lives "miraculously" improve on gluten-free diets are just properly treating their disease. In these cases, the transformative power of a gluten-free diet isn't a lie: it is a lifesaving scientific truth.

But that's where the transformative power of gluten-free stops. As far as we know, gluten is not toxic to the general population. It does not cause autism, or Alzheimer's, or ADHD. It does not give you wheat belly or grain brain, because there are no such things. Hoggan and

Gottschall were laypeople with axes to grind, so it makes sense they would demonize whatever caused their suffering. But how did 100 million Americans end up doing the same thing?

Why We Swallow the Gluten Lie

In the early 2000s, word began to spread about the evils of gluten-containing grains, particularly among sufferers of chronic health problems. The logic was simple and completely irrational, born of desperation: if a cure works miracles in one case, then it might in others. People trying to treat their own chronic health conditions—and those of their loved ones—came across theories like Hoggan's, which touted gluten-free diets as a solution for every health issue imaginable. The personal stories of Gottschall and Hoggan resonated, as did their distrust of stuck-up, hidebound doctors who offered no real help. Hopeful anecdotes circulated of children whose autism and learning disabilities had resolved on gluten-free diets—not an implausible occurrence, since undiagnosed CD can present with symptoms including headaches, numbness, seizures, poor mood, and behavioral disorders.

One of the most famous of these anecdotes came from former *Playboy* Playmate Jenny McCarthy. In 2004, McCarthy's young son, Evan, suffered a series of seizures and was diagnosed with autism. After an odyssey of visits to various doctors and hours spent on the "University of Google," McCarthy implemented a gluten-free, casein-free diet (casein is a protein commonly found in milk), and Evan got much, much better. McCarthy wrote about her experiences in a book, *Louder Than Words: A Mother's Journey in Healing Autism*, and the diet found a wider audience.

Meanwhile, diet gurus saw an opportunity to repackage the long-popular low carb Atkins diet using new myths and a new villain. In 2003, Internet sensation and naturopathic doctor Joseph Mercola published *The No-Grain Diet: Conquer Carbohydrate Addiction and*

Stay Slim for Life. Mercola—who opposes vaccination and has received numerous FDA warning letters—packed his book with speculations about the dangers of grains and gluten, especially to your waistline. Still in print, the book seriously misinforms the public about celiac disease and gluten sensitivity. ("Milder forms of celiac disease, referred to as 'gluten sensitivity,' affect about 15 percent of the population." False!) The myth of paradise past appears again, right down to the same sentence about grandparents that we saw in *Wheat Belly* and *Grain Brain*: "Unlike our grandparents, we can no longer take such things as a good night's sleep or clean, uncontaminated drinking water for granted."

All this was enough to get the ball rolling, but the popularity of gluten-free really exploded when sacred figures started to adopt the diet. No, not famous doctors: celebrities. There was celiac sufferer Elisabeth Hasselbeck, former cohost of *The View*, whose 2008 book *The G-Free Diet: A Gluten-Free Survival Guide* encouraged people without CD to go gluten-free. In the chapter "G-Free and Slim as Can Be!," Hasselbeck claims that a gluten-free diet is "beneficial for most [people]," and if she didn't have CD, she would still choose to be G-free. (The next chapter of the book is "The Autism Connection.") Jennifer Aniston went gluten-free in 2010, as part of a "baby-food diet" that prescribes fourteen portions of pureed foods a day followed by one normal dinner. The list of non-celiac gluten-free enthusiasts goes on: Oprah, Victoria Beckham, Gwyneth Paltrow, Miley Cyrus—all of whom implied that going gluten-free can be good for everyone. As Miley Cyrus tweeted: "everyone should try no gluten for a week! The change in your skin, physical and mental health is amazing! U won't go back!"

For scientists and physicians, however, tales of miracle diets are cause for cynicism, not celebration. When I ask Peter Gibson, coauthor of the Monash NCGS studies, about the relationship between gluten-free diets, weight loss, and general well-being, he has a different explanation—one that doesn't involve the elimination of a dietary villain.

"Much more likely is something I've noticed lots of times, even with family members," he says. "They've decided they're eating a lot of takeaway food, quick foods, not eating well at all. They read this thing about gluten-free, and then they're buying fresh vegetables, cooking well, and eating a lot better. Blaming the gluten is easy, but you could point to about a hundred things they're doing better."

Put simply: in some cases, eliminating gluten is just a proxy for cooking at home and cutting down on junk food. No one wants to cut down on foods they like. But when weight loss in itself is insufficient motivation, thinking that your favorite foods cause autism, foggy brain, and Alzheimer's can provide the boost you need to make good on your diet.

Experts like Gibson are also alert to the power of the placebo effect and the nocebo effect. The placebo effect occurs when expectation of benefit—not therapeutic value—produces positive results for a particular treatment. Acupuncture, painkillers, antidepressants, even some kinds of surgery: studies have shown that people respond well to fake versions of these interventions, reporting alleviated symptoms when the acupuncture needles don't pierce the skin, the pills are sugar, and the surgery is a sham.

The nocebo effect is the placebo effect in reverse. It was first documented when patients receiving sham pills ended up suffering negative side effects—because they expected the pills would make them feel bad. Now scientists recognize that nocebo effects must be taken into account when people report physiological food allergies. This applies even to people with documented allergies. One 2009 study of lactose found that 14 out of 54 patients with documented intolerance to lactose *reported symptoms after ingesting sugar pills.* They were lactose intolerant, but it was their expectation of symptoms that made them sick. Strong nocebo effects were also observed in the studies of gluten sensitivity out of Monash University.

Any analysis of gluten intolerance and gluten-free dieting must acknowledge the presence of substantial nocebo and placebo effects. With fears of gluten constantly reinforced in mainstream and social media, we should expect a significant nocebo reaction to gluten. Researchers do: in a 2013 review of the field, four experts on gluten wrote that although physiological non-celiac gluten sensitivity probably exists, at a prevalence of .063 to 6 percent of the general population, "in many circumstances non-celiac gluten sensitivity is an imaginary ailment that is caused by the nocebo effect of gluten ingestion." They also emphasized the likelihood that elimination diets would produce a placebo effect. Research suggests that placebo effects increase when the treatment is branded, expensive, and highly ritualized. Gluten-free diets—and most elimination diets—usually fit all of those criteria.

We've already seen the power of nocebo and placebo effects with MSG sensitivity, which should serve as a cautionary tale. As with MSG, the public's expectation of harm from gluten is fueled by highly profitable, unscientific fearmongering, validated by credentialed doctors. These doctors tap into deep-rooted worries about modernity and technology, identify a single cause of all our problems, and offer an easy solution. They spin stories of hidden killers and dietary miracles, and then they become merchants of false hope, healing problems they themselves have created.

MSG and gluten are not the same thing. I have said this before, but it bears constant repeating: unlike MSG, gluten threatens the health and lives of millions who have CD. While MSG sensitivity is almost entirely psychosomatic, the jury is still out on non-celiac gluten sensitivity. Anyone who says NCGS doesn't exist is as much a liar as the authors of *Wheat Belly* and *Grain Brain*. And though there's no doubt (one could say there's a *scientific consensus*) that Davis, Perlmutter, and their MSG-bashing forebears are irresponsible disgraces to the medical profession, Gottschall and Hoggan deserve our sympathy for their suffering and for their extraordinary efforts on behalf of others like them.

Yet we can't take our sympathy too far. Since gluten really is dangerous for some people, you may be tempted to give gluten-free alarmism a pass. Faddish celebrities and hyperbolic books have helped turn people's lives around and raised awareness of gluten intolerance. Sure, they distort the evidence and overstate the dangers of gluten. But is there any harm in that?

You bet there is.

When Lies Become Reality

"The Coca-Cola incident," as it is now referred to in the scientific literature, began on June 8, 1999, at a small school in Bornem, Belgium. Ten children fell mysteriously ill, and a staff inquiry determined the only feature held in common was their consumption of Coca-Cola that day. Equipped with just one school nurse, administrators sent the children to a local hospital and then reportedly visited classrooms asking if other children who had drunk Coke were feeling sick. The first ten children were joined by twenty-three more that evening, and another four the next morning. Symptoms included "abdominal discomfort, headache, nausea, malaise, respiratory problems, trembling, and dizziness." Once informed of the problem, Coca-Cola Belgium immediately recalled all bottles produced alongside those the children had consumed and issued a press release warning that Coke might produce headaches, nausea, and abdominal cramps.

At the time, Belgium was already reeling from another health scare known as "the dioxin crisis." In February of the same year, animal feed had been contaminated by dioxin, polychlorinated biphenyls, and dibenzofurans—all suspected carcinogens. The contamination remained secret until late May, when it was leaked to journalists, resulting in a massive recall of eggs, chicken, dairy, and meat. Outraged consumers, journalists, and activists engaged in a strident public debate about the safety of modern foods and chemicals.

This background set the stage for overreaction to new reports of food contamination. As one set of Belgian researchers, closely involved with the Coca-Cola incident, wrote in a retrospective account: "The dioxin crisis, therefore, combined a number of factors that are known to influence risk perception greatly, including outrage (against the failing authorities and against modern food production practices), dread (even minimal amounts of chemicals may damage health), and lack of control (the hazardous agent cannot be perceived)."

Print, radio, and television instantly drew parallels between the "Coca-Cola poisoning" and the dioxin crisis. Images of dead chickens were set side by side with images of soft drinks being destroyed. On June 11, Coca-Cola widened its product recall, and on June 14 the sale of all Coca-Cola products ceased throughout Belgium. Within twelve days of opening, a telephone help-line fielded 943 calls from symptomatic people.

But there was no contamination. Although Coca-Cola's internal investigation included toxicological data suggesting contamination via "bad carbon dioxide" and fungicides used on wooden transportation pallets, an independent, government-appointed committee concluded otherwise, finding absolutely no evidence whatsoever of any physiological reaction to Coca-Cola products. On July 3, the committee wrote a letter to the editor of the medical journal *The Lancet*: "The remarkable consistency of the reported complaints, as well as the context of anxiety and upheaval about the safety of modern foods, points to a diagnosis of mass sociogenic illness."

Mass sociogenic illness combines two kinds of lies: misinformation about external dangers (the Coke is poisoned), and self-deception about the effects of those dangers (the Coke is making me nauseated). It is a well-documented phenomenon, dating back to at least the fifteenth century, when groups of nuns who believed they were possessed by demons would imitate animals, bare their genitalia, shout expletives, and thrust their hips as if having intercourse. Demons no longer factor into most people's health concerns, so their role has been taken over by chemicals, bacteria, viruses, and the other invisible antagonists of modernity. In 1985, reports of exposure to nonexistent "toxic gas" produced chills, headaches, nausea, and breathlessness among students at a Singapore high school; the same occurred in 1998 at a high school in Tennessee, and variations continue to happen on a regular basis. That's the power of misinformation: even if you're drinking safe Coke or breathing clean air, rumors of illness can make you sick.

Another classic example of mass sociogenic illness is "wind turbine syndrome," which refers to the discredited theory that subaudible sound from wind turbines causes headaches and other adverse health effects. (The syndrome is widely publicized in English-speaking countries, where many people living near wind farms report symptoms. In countries with few English speakers, there are virtually no complaints.) To study the mechanism of wind turbine syndrome, a group of researchers from the University of Auckland primed one set of test subjects with literature that provoked high expectations of symptoms from infrasound exposure, and primed another set of subjects with literature that provoked low expectations. They then exposed both groups to infrasound and sham infrasound using a double-blind trial design, in which neither the subjects nor the researchers knew who was being exposed to the real thing. The subjects primed with high expectations reported a significant number of intense symptoms, independent of the authenticity of the infrasound. The low-expectancy group reported none.

"Expectations can cause symptoms," Keith Petrie, one of the coauthors, tells me. He compares wind turbine syndrome to medical students' disease, in which students are stricken with symptoms related to the conditions they are studying.

"Even the name you give to an illness has effects," says Petrie. "If you tell someone they have myalgic encephalomyelitis, they feel worse than if you tell them they have chronic fatigue syndrome. It sounds more medical, more real."

The effects described by Petrie are nocebo effects, and one way to think about mass sociogenic illness is as a large-scale nocebo effect. It stands to reason that alarmism about MSG, validated by newspaper articles and *60 Minutes*, was able create an epidemic of MSG sensitivity akin to mass sociogenic illness—and that the same could occur with other suspicious foodstuffs. In fact, Harvard physician and professor of medical sociology Nicholas Christakis has made this exact argument about peanut allergies. His 2008 opinion piece for the *British Medical Journal* is worth quoting in detail:

[It provokes] anxiety to imagine a hidden, deadly danger in so innocent a thing as having a snack in kindergarten. And being around others who are anxious heightens one's own anxiety. Seeing the concern about nut allergies in schools as a type of MPI [mass psychogenic/ sociogenic illness] is helpful in two ways. Firstly, the wholesale avoidance of nuts contributes to the problem by resulting in children who, lacking exposure to nuts, are actually sensitised to them. Through a feedback loop the policy of avoidance ends up creating the epidemic it is trying to stop. One recent UK study of more than 10,000 children documented that early exposure to peanuts reduces, not increases, the risk of allergy. Secondly, well-intentioned efforts to reduce exposure to nuts actually fan the flames, since they signal to parents that nuts are a clear and present danger. This encourages more parents to worry, which fuels the epidemic. It also encourages more parents to have their children tested, thus detecting mild and meaningless 'allergies' to nuts.

Mass sociogenic illness is real. Anxiety and negative expectations make people sick. These facts have profound implications for how we should view exaggerated accounts of the dangers posed by gluten and others foods. Recall the background sociological conditions that led to the Coca-Cola incident: outrage, dread, and lack of control. These are the key ingredients in alarmist accounts of gluten, whether in books, newspaper articles, or social media. Scientists and the government refuse to disclose the truth, we are told, because they are tainted by financial ties to industry. Gluten in even minimal amounts can cause addiction, weight gain, brain damage, cancer, Alzheimer's, and autism. You can't see it, but it will destroy you.

None of this denies the existence of celiac disease or the possibility of non-celiac gluten sensitivity. Hyperbolic fearmongering, however, makes it difficult to distinguish those who suffer physiological reactions from those whose symptoms are caused by expectations of ill health, reinforced by outrage at Big Food and Big Pharma and dread of modernity.

Moreover, it is foolish not to consider the possibility that some milder reactions to gluten are created or exacerbated by repeated exposure to distortions and outright lies of the sort found in *Dangerous Grains*, *Wheat Belly*, and *Grain Brain*, amplified in the hysterical echo chamber of news outlets and social media. Nausea, headaches, and dizziness are no less worrisome if they are induced by books and articles instead of pills—and we should guard against the side effects of dangerous lies and misrepresentations just as we do against the side effects of dangerous medicine.

"Diet" Is a Four-Letter Word

Encouraging the general public to eliminate gluten from their diet, especially by associating it with weight gain, has another potentially lethal side effect: eating disorders. Lifetime prevalence estimates in Americans of anorexia, bulimia, and binge eating disorder are 0.9, 1.5, and 3.5 percent among women, and 0.3, 0.5, and 2.0 percent among men. All who suffer from eating disorders have a significantly increased risk of death, and anorexia and bulimia are particularly deadly, with a mortality rate of around 4 percent. There are easily ten times more yearly deaths from eating disorders in the United States than from *all food allergies combined*.

Bombarded with headlines that read "Gluten Confirmed to Cause Serious Weight Gain" and "Three Hidden Ways That Wheat Makes You Fat," the average dieter will surely be tempted by a gluten-free approach to weight loss. I asked specialists if these approaches concern them.

"Any restrictive diet puts a vulnerable person at risk," says Dr. Edward Tyson, whose private practice in Austin, Texas, focuses specifically on eating disorders. "Ninety-five percent of my patients start with some kind of food that's taboo. Thirty years ago it was mostly fat. Then Atkins with carbohydrates. Now it's sugar, processed foods, and gluten."

Disordered eaters usually start off restricting just one food, out of concern for their health or their weight. But the logic of food restriction is slippery. If we haven't evolved to eat gluten, then, as *Wheat Belly* and *Grain Brain* tell us, we also haven't evolved to eat grains. Nor, for that matter, should we eat anything processed, artificial, or unnatural, words so vague that a person prone to disordered eating is soon at a loss to find any safe food.

"By the time they come to me, they've eliminated everything," Tyson says. "Lactose, carbs, gluten, my gosh, all kinds of things. And since they're afraid of losing control, if they even try to eat one of those foods it's scary, it's failure."

Jennifer J. Thomas, assistant professor of psychology at Harvard Medical School and codirector of the Eating Disorders Clinical and Research Program at Massachusetts General Hospital, confirms that she encounters the same pattern.

"There are no studies, but anecdotally we see this all the time," she tells me. "Of course most of my patients are reading these types of books, and it definitely concerns me. People typically can't stick to these rigid diets. They start to crave the foods they've eliminated, and then the eating disorder gets worse because they start bingeing on the very foods they're trying to get rid of."

Thomas also points out how psychological factors can produce the same symptoms as physiological reactions to food.

"Look at the criteria for panic attacks or other anxiety disorders," she says. "Panic makes you feel like you're going to have diarrhea, or going to vomit. Fear of demonized foods can cause these reactions."

Anxiety about food produces physical symptoms. And while one way to control those symptoms is by eliminating the source of anxiety— gluten, fat, sugar, MSG—another approach is to eliminate the myths and lies responsible for making those foods anxiety-inducing in the first place.

That's a difficult task when fearmongers are everywhere. Before coming to her, many of Thomas's patients visit traditional doctors to get tested for suspected allergies, and one of the most common is gluten sensitivity. If the test results for celiac disease come back negative, it can be the start of an eating disorder nightmare.

"They'll go to someone else, a non-MD allergist, and get a print-out of literally dozens, if not hundreds, of foods they can't eat," says Thomas. "There's hardly anything left."

According to Tyson and Thomas, dieters often rationalize their food fears with so-called lifestyle diets. When fat was taboo, vegetarianism or veganism provided the supporting framework for its elimination. Now they are seeing more of the Paleolithic diet, with its evolutionary arguments against consumption of gluten-containing wheat as well as other "dangerous grains."

Both Tyson and Thomas are careful to point out that most lifestyle dieters, whether vegan, Paleo, or gluten-free, do *not* develop eating disorders.

"Eating disorders have always been around, with or without these fads," says Thomas. "But I still believe these diets can be a gateway to an eating disorder, and that they can help you maintain it. It used to be socially acceptable to say you're on a diet, but not anymore. Diet is a four-letter word. Nowadays people will worry that you have an eating disorder if you say, 'I'm afraid of getting fat,' but they won't bat an eyelash if you say you're Paleo or gluten-free."

The suggestion that elimination diets can function, *in some cases*, as an excuse for restricted eating is offensive to many lifestyle dieters, but there is growing acknowledgment of the problem. One courageous person raising awareness is Amy Kubal, "the Paleo Dietitian," a licensed dietitian who has worked in the Paleo community for more than a decade. In February 2014, Amy came out on a prominent Paleo website as anorexic.

> **"People will worry that you have an eating disorder if you say, 'I'm afraid of getting fat,' but they won't bat an eyelash if you say you're Paleo or gluten-free."**

"In my case," she wrote, "Paleo was a convenient way to *justify* restriction. I entered the eating disorder world with an intense fear of fat, a fear that didn't go away with Paleo—it let up a little but it also villainized many of the foods that were once 'safe' to me. Now carbs, dairy, beans, grains, and fat were evil and my list kept getting longer."

Amy spoke candidly with me about her own experience and her impression of the Paleo community in general.

"You know, it works for some people," she says. "But for 60 to 70 percent, it turns into a religion. Following this is like their commandment—does that have gluten? Does this? Their lives revolve around it, thinking constantly about what foods are at the places they're going to be. I have more and more clients who bring their own food to restaurants and family gatherings."

The more we talked, the more frustrated Amy got—at people's unwillingness to acknowledge the problem, and the effect it had on her own life and the lives of people she cared about.

"It's a secret. It's the elephant in the room," she tells me. "A year ago I weighed probably seventy-two pounds. Nobody said anything. Nobody! I went to a naturopath who was supposed to help me, and she put me on a cleanse. A fucking cleanse! I was taking shit out when I needed to be putting stuff back in."

Part of the problem is that people like her start thinking they have reactions to food, which makes it impossible to "put stuff back in." She, too, had gone to a nontraditional allergist and been diagnosed with celiac disease—without so much as a blood test.

"No more gluten after that. Then I talked myself into being sensitive to nuts. And then I talked myself into not being able to handle dairy. And when you tell yourself those things, it's a self-fulfilling prophecy."

Amy is no longer sensitive to dairy or nuts. Working with an eating disorder specialist, she made up her mind that dairy wasn't actually going to harm her.

"He told me to go out and try it," she says. "And I'll be goddamned—it didn't make me sick. Honestly, I hope gluten is the same way for me. I hope I've just spun myself up around it, and it's going to be okay."

Test First, Test Right

The risk of having a misdiagnosis—or a self-diagnosis—turn into a physical disorder isn't limited to gluten sensitivity and food allergies. Nortin Hadler, rheumatologist and professor at the University of North Carolina School of Medicine, has spent much of his career criticizing how everyday symptoms—acne, headaches, fatigue, wrinkles, joint pain—get turned into medical conditions. This medicalization leads to anxiety, increased pain, useless diets, and unnecessary medical procedures. Hadler cuts through the traditional dogma that "conventional" physicians just want to pump you full of drugs and perform surgery. In *Worried Sick: A Prescription for Health in an Overtreated America*, he argues against *all overdiagnosis*, whether by diet gurus or your general practitioner.

"Diagnostic workups and labeling are very dangerous," he warns me. "They shift your self-image, and that's true whether you come to me or a naturopath. These visits are not trivial events. When you try out a treatment, you aren't just accepting the potion, you're accepting the notion of the potion."

For Hadler, Amy Kubal's story would represent a tremendous victory, an instance where the courage to question one's diagnosis led to a cure. But such stories are few and far between. The shift in self-image that attends a diagnosis is very difficult to reverse. Eating disorder specialists like Edward Tyson and Jennifer Thomas work with their patients one-on-one for hours, cultivating trust and openness. There's no other way to show someone that their identity, their faith in themselves and their costly dietary ritual, was misplaced.

"Asking someone to question their relationship to a food they've eliminated, it's like asking someone to change religions," says Tyson. "I have to be very careful, and it takes a long time."

> **"Asking someone to question their relationship to a food they've eliminated, it's like asking someone to change religions."**

Tyson is right to be cautious. Even with mass sociogenic illness, waltzing in and shouting, "Don't worry, it was all in your head!" isn't a particularly effective strategy. Simon Wessely, a psychiatrist and expert on mass sociogenic illness, urges thoughtfulness in responses to situations like the Coca-Cola incident.

"A firm public message that certain symptoms are probably psychological in origin will probably help prevent their spread," he wrote for the *New England Journal of Medicine*, "but possibly at the cost of alienating those already affected and their families. The challenge is to convey the scientific reality without being seen as blaming or demeaning the victims."

Needless to say, that is my challenge as well.

Look, science does not have all the answers. What appears psychosomatic can actually be physiological—the sad truth for millions of undiagnosed celiac sufferers. Tragically, the history of medicine is filled with examples of physiological conditions that received mistaken psychological diagnoses. Multiple sclerosis, long thought extremely rare, was routinely identified as hysteria throughout the first half of the twentieth century. Without a doubt the future will yield further examples of the same.

Yet the existence of misdiagnosed physiological conditions does not mean we should dismiss the possibility of mass sociogenic gluten sensitivity. It does not mean there is no such thing as placebo and nocebo effects. And it does not mean we should trust charlatans and fearmongers, whose stock-in-trade is whipping up antiestablishment resentment—using studies produced by that very establishment!—and then cashing in on the panic they create.

In truth, Perlmutter and Davis are the ones pretending that science has all the answers. The established experts on CD, on the other hand, are willing to admit uncertainty. It is they, not the "maverick" diet gurus, who exemplify the caution, rigor, and humility that resulted in Dicke's discovery of a gluten-free treatment for CD, and it is they who produce genuine medical advances.

Most people don't have the time to read hundreds of peer-reviewed studies or interview specialists. When people like Perlmutter and Davis fill their books with scientific citations, they effectively camouflage their true identities. Fortunately, there's another way to identify false prophets: just compare how they talk with past peddlers of miracle cures. When you do, you'll find that not much has changed. Like faith healers, proponents of early-twentieth-century dietary regimens would testify to their near instantaneous life-changing power, often starting with their personal conversion story. In the words of food historian Harvey Levenstein: "[They] would tell of their own devastating health problems, miraculously cured by the proposed diet—mysterious or common physical or psychological ailments that had defied the greatest of modern medical minds had disappeared once certain foods were added or deleted from the diet."

Dr. William Davis, the author of *Wheat Belly*, made just these sorts of faith-revival-style claims for his own dietary regimen in a recent radio debate:

> You have a drop in weight, you have relief from rheumatoid arthritis, you have a drop in multiple autoimmune diseases, you have a reduction in asthma, you have a drop in psychiatric illness. Yes, you could

use it as a diet, you could use it as a weight-loss tool [. . .] but you also see transformations in health. I've seen [. . .] people come back from the brink of near death, and I'm not exaggerating when I say that. People who throw away their wheelchairs, crutches, and walkers. People who throw away insulin and three diabetic drugs, throw away three drugs for rheumatoid arthritis, their two inhalers for asthma.

This is predatory marketing at its worst, the promise of miracles to those who are sick and vulnerable. Not only that, when people "try out" gluten-free diets, as Davis and other gluten-free enthusiasts suggest they should, they delegitimize the very real disease that so many celiac sufferers are dealing with. Going gluten-free isn't fun. It isn't a new way to lose weight. It isn't what evolution tells us to do. There's no conclusive evidence that it prevents cancer, Alzheimer's, autism, or whatever it is that you fear most. It can lead to eating disorders, and it can cause you to start manifesting symptoms that didn't exist before.

That's why you should listen to the experts, the ones who don't spread anxiety about modernity or promise miracles. Dr. Peter Green, director of the Celiac Disease Center at Columbia University Medical Center, calls on all people who suspect gluten sensitivity to go to a doctor and get tested. Celiac disease is genetic, he points out. If you have it, then family members need to know. Other specialists agree.

So does Priyanka Chugh, health advocate, aspiring physician, and creator of the blog *The Adventures of Anti-Wheat Girl*. Ten years ago, Priyanka's then six-year-old brother, Pranav, presented with classic CD symptoms: abnormally short stature, weight loss, and gastrointestinal problems. He was lucky—Priyanka's mother is a pediatric gastroenterologist, and she immediately recognized the symptoms as linked to dietary difficulties. After a battery of tests, the young boy was diagnosed with celiac disease and quickly improved on a gluten-free diet.

At the time, twelve-year-old Priyanka didn't look like a celiac sufferer. She was tall and slightly overweight, without any behavioral or
digestive issues. But because her brother had CD, the whole family got
tested. Though neither her sister, Prajnika, nor her parents tested positive, Priyanka did. (Her family continues to get tested on a yearly basis,
since CD develops when as-yet-unknown environmental factors "trig-
ger" a genetic predisposition.)

"If my brother had never been diagnosed, I would never have been
diagnosed," she tells me. "You definitely have a responsibility to your
family."

Priyanka also worries that people who go gluten-free without re-
alizing they have CD may underestimate the seriousness of their condition.

"If you don't have this strict reason to be gluten-free, then you may
cheat," she says. "That's extremely dangerous. And you also might not
get tested for other conditions, like diabetes or osteoporosis, which
often occur alongside celiac disease."

So if you suspect gluten sensitivity, get tested for celiac disease: for
yourself, for your family, and for the sake of the greater community
of celiac sufferers who don't want the seriousness of their condition
diminished. And "test right," as Dr. Joseph Murray of the Mayo Clinic
put it in an interview. Don't depend on an unapproved diagnostic tool,
like the opinion of a naturopathic doctor or the popular Cyrex Array
tests recommended by Dr. Perlmutter. Why not? Just ask Dr. Alessio
Fasano:

> When you develop a new drug or test, there are these rules created
> by the American Medical Association that [we are asked] to obey. We
> don't take this lightly since we are dealing with health and therefore
> the well-being of human beings, so we want to make sure that we do
> this right. If somebody will develop a new tool, a new biomarker, a

new test—first and foremost, it needs to be validated. The tests that are offered for gluten sensitivity didn't go through this vigorous validation process.

Test first, test right. And if you don't have celiac disease, don't assume mainstream medicine has failed you. Instead, consider the possibility that your fear of gluten is just the latest in a long line of groundless dietary paranoias, based on nothing more than myth and superstition, spoiling your favorite foods and putting you at risk for eating disorders.

After all, that's exactly what fear of fat turned out to be.

CHAPTER THREE

Fat Magic

Why Did Denmark Tax the Danish?

For decades, "low fat" has been synonymous with heart health and weight loss. In order to live longer and shed pounds, millions of consumers compromise on their best-loved foods. Fat-free yogurt. "Skinny" lattes. Turkey bacon. Grocery store aisles are packed with alternative versions of fatty favorites and we choke them down, even though they don't taste as good. Food companies spend millions each year trying (and failing) to close the quality gap between low-fat and regular versions of treats, using "ice-structuring proteins" cloned from Arctic fish to improve the "mouthfeel" of reduced-fat ice cream (Unilever), or special batters that prevent french fries from absorbing cooking oil (Burger King).

If you've done your homework and consulted the authorities, sacrificing high-fat pleasure for low-fat health seems like it makes good sense. The American Heart Association advises us to consume only fat-free or low-fat milk, vegetables "without added fat," lean cuts of

pork loin, and skinless chicken breasts. Cooks should use low-fat peanut butter and swap regular butter for cooking sprays (with "butter
flavor"). Doing so, they say, will help prevent heart disease and keep
off extra weight.

Though the AHA frowns on too much of any fat, saturated fats—
so-called because the fat molecules are "saturated" with hydrogen
atoms—are identified as convicted killers. "Decades of sound science,"
reads the AHA's website, "has proven [saturated fats] can raise your
'bad' cholesterol and raise your risk for heart disease." There is simply
no room for doubt: for the American Heart Association, the science on
saturated fat is rock-solid, like your arteries after a year of eating too
much bacon.

The AHA is wrong. That's *not* what decades of sound science has
proven. It's what decades of loud public policy makers have said—and,
unfortunately, public policy doesn't always proceed from sound science. The closest we have come to a truly unanimous consensus on fat
is that if you eat an excessive amount of calories, you will gain weight,
and fat has lots of calories in it. But
we're nowhere near that kind of
certainty when it comes to pin-
pointing the effects of saturated fat
on heart disease, or even the effects
of a high-fat diet on obesity rates.
The AHA, for instance, does not
mention a 2012 study published in
the *American Journal of Clinical
Nutrition* that suggests saturated
fat from dairy may *reduce* risk of
cardiovascular disease, while saturated fat from red meat seems to increase it. Nor does it mention a 2013 study published in the *Annals of
Internal Medicine*, which called into question the wisdom of reducing

> **The closest we have
> come to a truly
> unanimous consensus
> on fat is that if you eat
> an excessive amount of
> calories, you will gain
> weight, and fat has
> lots of calories in it.**

saturated fat. "Current evidence," wrote the study's authors, "does not clearly support cardiovascular guidelines that encourage high consumption of polyunsaturated fatty acids and low consumption of total saturated fats." Evidently the American Heart Association thinks sound science involves ignoring legitimate controversy over its chosen dietary guidelines.

Despite scientific uncertainty, dogmatic anti-fat rhetoric is so persuasive that an entire nation recently levied a "sin tax" on saturated fats, the same kind of tax paid on cigarettes and alcohol. Danes are comparatively healthy and svelte—only 13.4 percent of the country is obese, compared with 35.9 percent of the United States. Nevertheless, Danish policy makers felt that precautionary measures were necessary, and in 2011 they levied the world's first tax on saturated fat. Citizens had to cough up extra cash for most products that contained more than 2.3 percent saturated fat, including various cooking oils, butter, cheese, bacon, sausage, and lard. Prices also rose for prepared foods containing those ingredients such as pizza, butter cookies, and, of course, Danish pastries.

Instead of decrying the tax as a premature move based on speculative science, high-profile public health advocates in America applauded it as a courageous step toward curbing rising rates of obesity and associated chronic disease. "Let us congratulate Denmark on what could be viewed as a revolutionary experiment," wrote Marion Nestle, professor of nutrition, food studies, and public health at New York University. "I can't wait to see the results."

The results were surely disappointing. Infuriated Danes began crossing the border to buy forbidden fats in Germany and Sweden, and only a year later the Danish tax ministry announced they would be repealing the fat tax.

Danish government officials would have been justified in attempting the fat tax if saturated fat really did pose a tremendous public health risk, like tobacco. Indeed, Nestle and other advocates of the tax

explained its potential benefits with analogies to tobacco. Their rationale was straightforward: cigarettes are subject to successful sin taxes
across the globe. Cigarette smoke clogs our lungs and causes cancer;
saturated fat clogs our bodies with excess bulk and causes chronic disease. Both are undeniable threats to public health and call for extreme
preventative action. The political wisdom of the fat tax might have
been uncertain, but, to the Danish government and international public health advocates, the science behind it was clear.

Except the science wasn't clear, not by a long shot, and it never has
been.

It's All a Big Fat Lie

Since the 1960s, scientists and journalists have been questioning the
conventional wisdom that consumption of saturated fats—banished
to the tip of the food pyramid in the increasingly obese US—will
make you fat and kill you. But for a long time, these dissenting voices
remained largely ignored. Intense public and political vilification of
saturated fats obscured the scientific community's uncertainty. Fearmongering was rampant. In 1965, newspapers quoted Harvard nutritionist Jean Mayer blasting low-carb diets, which, because they led
to increased fat consumption, were "in a sense, equivalent to mass
murder." In only a few decades, Americans, and eventually much of
the world, came to fear fatty meat and butter nearly as much as they
feared cigarettes.

Slowly but surely, the ridiculousness of comparing low-carb diets
to mass murder and saturated fat to tobacco inspired skeptics to become more vocal. Most prominent among them was American science
journalist Gary Taubes, who documented and publicized the controversy's history. In two articles, "The Soft Science of Dietary Fat" and
"What If It's All Been a Big Fat Lie?," Taubes made a compelling case
that no one actually knew the dietary causes of cardiovascular disease

and obesity. Saturated fat, he argued, was nothing more than a convenient scapegoat, and a modern one at that.

Taubes followed up his articles with an influential book, *Good Calories, Bad Calories*, in which he laid the blame for obesity and heart disease on carbohydrates, not fat. While his thesis about what causes weight gain remains highly controversial—Taubes himself admits it requires further evidence—his case against the demonization of saturated fats was right on target. Replacing saturated fats with carbohydrates did nothing to improve rates of cardiovascular disease, and studies confirmed that Dr. Atkins and his followers weren't crazy: high-fat diets were no worse than low-fat diets for losing weight in the long term, and might be more effective during the initial phase of dieting. Saturated fats could no longer be painted as a perfect dietary villain.

You'd think all scientists and policy makers would just admit to uncertainty about the danger of saturated fat, instead of doubling down on that belief. But there's still evidence of a deep-seated bias, one that appears insensitive to evidence and unwilling to acknowledge controversy. Staring at a June 2014 *Time* magazine cover featuring the simple, sensationalist imperative, *Eat Butter*, many nutrition scientists explained that although saturated fat may have been excessively demonized, it still qualifies as a minor demon. Harvard physician and nutrition researcher Walter Willett told CNN that "heart-healthy" plant-based oils like olive oil are certainly better for you than butter. And in a series of blistering opinion pieces for the Huffington Post, Yale's Dr. David Katz argued that proponents of a low-fat, high-plant diet were never *really* wrong. It's just that instead of embracing olives and kale, Americans went and traded saturated fat for garbage, in what Katz calls a giant collective turn to SnackWell's cookies. Was it a mistake to vilify saturated fats? Probably—we "were almost certainly silly to do so," he says—but then again, probably not.

"We have very compelling evidence," writes Katz, usually a level-headed opponent of dogmatic dietary advice, "regarding the kinds of foods and diets that are associated with reduced risk of premature death and chronic disease—and they are not diets high in saturated fat!" With similar confidence, the American Institute for Cancer Research declares on its website that "many major studies show that people who follow plant-based diets [. . .] are leaner, lead healthier lives, have lower rates of mortality, and lower risk for many cancers and other chronic diseases."

Yet the AICR's preferred studies are far from the last word. Scientific certainty about what leads to leaner, healthier living is unjustified. Let's start with "leaner." Legions of Atkins and Paleo dieters—as well as obesity experts—fiercely contest the superiority of a plant-based diet for making you "leaner." Like all nutrition science, the science of weight loss is complicated and uncertain. The relative effectiveness of moderate exercise, long thought a key component in reducing obesity rates, is now under scrutiny. (A recent editorial in the *International Journal of Epidemiology* is titled "Physical activity does not influence obesity risk: time to clarify the public health message.") Even the wisdom of gradual weight loss is questionable, in light of a new study that suggests crash dieters don't gain back weight any more than dieters who drop pounds gradually. While nearly everyone agrees that reducing calories is essential to weight loss, the best way to do so remains hotly debated, which is why well-regarded bariatric doctors like Canada's Yoni Freedhoff, author of *The Diet Fix*, argue that the "best way" to get lean is simply the way that works for you, sustainably, over the long term.

So much for low-fat diets making you "leaner." What about "healthier"? Here, too, the science is uncertain: we just don't know the role that saturated fat plays in heart disease. While Dr. Dean Ornish has produced studies suggesting the efficacy of a low-fat vegan diet for reversing heart disease, his regimen also entails radical lifestyle modifications, including an hour of daily stress-management techniques. Without controlling for the benefits of meditation and weekly group counseling sessions, there's no way to prove that Ornish's dietary recommendations alone lead to better heart health.

Absent decisive evidence, it's a mistake to condemn saturated fat. In the October 2013 *British Medical Journal*, cardiologist Aseem Malhotra stated flat-out that physicians should stop connecting heart health with diets low in animal fat. "Recent cohort studies," wrote Malhotra, "have not supported any significant association between saturated fat intake and cardiovascular disease."

Malhotra's editorial prompted strong objections from British policymakers. Alison Tedstone, director of diet and obesity at Public Health England, said the "government's advice is based on a wealth of evidence. . . . The *BMJ* article is based on opinion, rather than a complete review of the research." Malhotra disagreed. "From the analysis of the independent evidence that I have done," he said, "saturated fat from nonprocessed food is not harmful and probably beneficial. Butter, cheese, yoghurt, and eggs are generally healthy and not detrimental."

In short, there is no consensus on the optimal amount of fat consumption—and type of fat—for weight loss and heart health. That's to be expected. Uncertainty and skepticism should be the default positions in nutrition science. Studying the link between diet, weight, and disease is incredibly difficult, and truly representative controlled studies are impossible. (*Okay, half of this country will eat lots of butter for thirty years, and the other half will be vegan. And the study will be blinded. Neither half will know what they're eating!*) Denmark did not have a solid basis for its fat tax, and Harvard nutritionists don't have enough evidence to warrant instructing people to "limit butter," as they do in their new "healthy eating plate." Eating butter may lead to cardiovascular disease—or it may not. We just don't know. The same is true for weight loss. Currently, the only proven way to control one's weight is by eating in moderation. Low fat, low carb, low *whatever*: for successful dieting, the common denominator is *lower* consumption across the board. Research has yet to substantiate targeting fat or carbohydrates. Period, end of story. Anyone who tells you otherwise is probably trying to sell you on the diet that worked for them—or the dietary advice upon which they've built their livelihood.

Okay. Eating fat doesn't necessarily make you fat or sick. Yet public health officials continue to evangelize a diet low in saturated fat, without so much as a disclaimer about the highly speculative nature of the recommendation. Health-conscious consumers still opt for low-fat ice cream and pretend to prefer turkey bacon. Is this persistent anti-fat bias a product of bad science, or is something more going on?

The Scapegoat

In Taubes's *Good Calories, Bad Calories* and journalist Nina Teicholz's *The Big Fat Surprise*, the story of how we came to fear fat starts in the mid-twentieth century with a nutrition scientist named Ancel Keys. Teicholz paints a damning portrait of Keys as power-hungry, arrogant, and ruthless, the kind of researcher who develops a theory and then sticks to it, no matter what the evidence says. "All of the ailments that have been ascribed to eating fat over the years," writes Teichholz, "not just heart disease but also obesity, cancer, diabetes, and more—stem from the implantation of this idea in the nutrition establishment by Ancel Keys and his perseverance in promoting it."

Taubes agrees. He maintains that prior to the 1950s, pretty much everyone knew obesity resulted from excess carbohydrate consumption. To prove the point, his book opens with a discussion of William Banting, a British undertaker whose 1863 *Letter on Corpulence* became a best-selling diet manual. According to Taubes, Banting's strategy was almost identical to that of Dr. Atkins and other latter-day low-carb advocates. "[Banting] ate three meals a day of meat, fish, or game, usually five or six ounces at a meal, with an ounce or two of stale toast or cooked fruit on the side. He had his evening tea with a few more ounces of fruit or toast. He scrupulously avoided any other food that might contain either sugar or starch, in particular bread, milk, sweets, beer, and potatoes."

But in his eagerness to demonstrate the historical ubiquity of low-carb diets, Taubes omits a central feature of Banting's approach: it was also low fat. An early-twentieth-century diet book, *How to Get Thin and How to Acquire Plumpness*, remarks that Banting's diet required "the removal, as far as possible, of all saccharine, starchy, *and fatty foods*" [my emphasis added]. Banting forbade butter and cream, and in his appendix he writes that dieters would do well to omit pork "for its fattening character," and salmon, herring, and eel, "owing to their oily nature."

Clearly there is more to anti-fat bias than Ancel Keys. Taubes and Teicholz write as if contemporary fear of fat resulted from a twentieth-century triumph of bad science over conventional dietary wisdom. But Keys's research can't explain why Banting and his contemporaries also thought eating fat made you fat.

The reality is that Banting, Keys, the Danish government, the American Heart Association, and most Americans have come under the influence of age-old magical thinking. When people buy nasty ice cream and watery yogurt and lean bison meat in hopes of losing weight, they are actually buying into an ancient, potent myth, enshrined in a familiar cliché: *You are what you eat*.

We ignore the historical influence of this myth at our own peril. Like holy texts, the literature of nutrition science is vast, vague, and highly contested, making it easy to cherry-pick whatever data confirm your biases. If we want to get over our fear of fat and start making rational dietary choices, the solution isn't running more studies. It's to recognize *you are what you eat* for what it is—and then stop believing in fat magic.

Why Magic Makes Sense

In early 2014, a bizarre Chinese criminal case briefly captured the attention of Western media outlets. Authorities in the city of Qinzhou had arrested one Mr. Xu, a real estate developer, and several accomplices for purchasing and slaughtering three tigers. According to the prosecutor, Mr. Xu had "a quirky appetite for eating tiger penis and drinking tiger blood." He was tried along with fourteen other defendants and a tiger smuggler, all of whom pleaded guilty to killing more than ten tigers over the past several years.

To people unfamiliar with traditional Chinese medicine, an appetite for tiger penis might seem quirky. But the prosecutor should have known better. Mr. Xu's culinary choices reflect a long-standing tradition that continues to grieve conservationists and animal rights activists. Ten years earlier, the *New York Times* ran an article about dwindling tiger and rhinoceros populations in Africa and Vietnam that explains Mr. Xu's motives perfectly. The populations were shrinking because poachers were killing the animals to sell their bones, flesh, horns, and blood to Taiwan, Hong Kong, China, and Singapore. Demand was due to a powerful myth: "In the reductionist view of Chinese medical practitioners, you are what you eat. Tiger eyes are said to improve vision; a tiger penis boiled in soup brings virility. . . . The succulent meat of a bear's paw is said to give strength."

Belief that you absorb the physical—and moral—qualities of your food is a near universal superstition.

Belief that you absorb the physical—and moral—qualities of your food is a near universal superstition. In *The Golden Bough*, the great theorist of magic James Frazer famously catalogs endless dietary rules based on "sympathetic magic," or the idea that an effect resembles its cause. Native Americans believed that eating venison made you fleet of foot, while eating clumsy bears, helpless dunghill fowls, and the "heavy wallowing swine" made you slower, both physically and mentally. In Turkey, children slow to speak were fed bird tongues. Traditional Zulu doctors prescribed the ground bones of old cows so their patients might absorb longevity. To jump higher, Northern Australian aborigines ate kangaroo and emu. The Mishing people of India fed tiger to men as a means of fortifying their strength, but not to women, for fear "it would make them too strong-minded."

In some ways, magical thinking is more like science than religious faith. Magic is governed by simple and intuitively plausible laws that explain the natural world without supernatural forces: beet juice is red, blood is red, therefore drinking beet juice ought to replenish blood. It makes so much sense—but is totally incorrect. Believing that beet juice turns into blood is simply bad science, in the same way that believing in paradise past is bad history.

Admittedly there are rare instances when *you are what you eat* is true. Eating too many carrots really can turn your skin yellowish, a condition known as carotenemia. But there are also instances when psychics' predictions come true. *You are what you eat* is superstition, not science, no matter how plausible it seems. The Chinese market for tiger penis is shrinking now that Viagra has been introduced. But since no Viagra has been invented for weight loss, the market for low-fat products is still strong.

We need to recognize our fear of fat for what it really is. Otherwise *you are what you eat* will continue to derail nutrition science, inspire bad public policy, and, worst of all, force people to continue eating turkey bacon, skim-milk lattes, and Edy's Slow Churned Ice Cream.

Eat Fat, Get Fat

Translated into a theory about what makes people fat, *you are what eat* becomes: *If you eat animal fat, you will become fat.* And indeed, since the beginning of recorded medicine, that's exactly what we see. Writing in the second century CE, the Greek physician Galen distinguished three kinds of fat people: chubby, fat, and obese. Since obesity limited one's ability to walk, reach, breathe, bathe, and give birth, he felt it necessitated medical intervention. To slim down obese patients, Galen prescribed a combination of exercise (including jogging), massage, and a special diet. Obese people, said Galen, should only eat the meat of wild animals, ideally mountain dwellers. Milk and cheese are forbidden, along with "animals' brains, intestines, liver, spleen, and kidneys." Plant bulbs and snails are also proscribed.

You are what you eat is clearly hard at work in Galen's dietary recommendations. Wild animals are leaner than domesticated ones, and those that live on mountains are leaner still. Eat lean, stay lean. Eat fat, get fat. Plant bulbs are bulbous, so if you eat them you'll become bulbous yourself. Snails resemble fatty tissue—better not add them to your own fatty tissue. Of course, Galen himself didn't recognize these recommendations as superstitious. Instead, he used the medical science of the time—which involved four bodily fluids called "humors"—to rationalize his magical thinking. (For example, he theorized that obesity was caused by "excess blood," and valley animals were fattening because of their "wet temperament.")

The myth of *you are what you eat* continued to influence nutrition science long after Galen. During the early Renaissance, doctors claimed that red grapes were "good for the blood." The Italian gastronomist Platina asserted that pork caused gluttony, and justified his conclusion using the language of humoral medicine: pork was "excessively humid." But sympathetic magic provided the logic—pigs are gluttonous, so you'll absorb their gluttonous nature if you eat them.

During this time, *you are what you eat* also made people think that fat *inside* the body behaves the same way as fat *outside* the body. The physician Erastus, for instance, argued in 1580 that cold temperatures facilitated the formation of human fat. As food historian Ken Albala points out, Erastus assumes continuity between the properties of fatty tissue and "the properties of butter and other fats outside the body, which are liquid if hot but solid at colder temperatures." Scarily, we haven't come too far since Erastus. The metaphor of "melting" body fat is still common in the rhetoric of diet and exercise programs. Though completely inaccurate, the intuitive sensibility of this metaphor is so powerful that literal versions persist today. Diet books tout foods as fat burners, and quacks market lasers that will "literally melt fat." The fat-melting lasers are an updated version of a treatment by twentieth-century French medical consultant Dr. Laissus, who locked fat patients in a box lined with electric lightbulbs and subjected them to intense heat of up to 60 degrees Celsius (140 degrees Fahrenheit).

As seventeenth-century doctors and scientists developed creative new approaches to obesity, *you are what you eat* remained as powerful as ever. Johann Friedrich Held, the first person to define obesity according to belt size (thirty-six inches), prescribed a unique battery of purgatives, emetics, and sudorifics (sweat-inducing herbs) that he felt would speed food and fluids through the body. He also believed that salt was useful for "drying" up fat, and recommended that obese people consume cured meats. But, in keeping with *you are what you eat*, Held inveighed against fatty meat. Humoral medicine was no longer in vogue, so Held theorized that fatty foods are difficult to digest and therefore accumulate more quickly in the body. The scientific language he used to rationalize the myth had changed, but the myth itself remained the same.

Though morbid obesity had been treated as a cause for medical concern since at least the time of Galen, eighteenth-century England witnessed an explosion of interest in the condition. Historian Lucia Dacome chronicles how British consumer society faced rising obesity rates, which were reflected in popular alarmism that foreshadowed present-day complaints. Thomas Short, in his 1727 treatise, *A Discourse Concerning the Causes and Effects of Corpulency*, lamented that "no Age did ever afford more Instances of Corpulency than our own." To counter this disastrous trend, Short recommended unusual remedies like wearing flannel shirts and moving from marshy areas. Yet he never abandoned the intuitively plausible logic of *you are what you eat*. In addition to recommending moving from marshes, Short told obese people to avoid fatty meats, particularly veal, pork, bacon, lamb, and mutton, in favor of fish and fowl.

Short's approach to weight loss may have worked for some, but it wasn't because they avoided fatty meats and marshes. It wasn't because they drank "Water a little acidulated with Vinegar, or Juice of Lemons," a habit that some dieters embrace today, perhaps without knowing about its origin in the belief that acidic liquids help wash the fat out of your body. No, any success was due to Short's time-honored advice of eating a "moderate, spare" diet—the same pedestrian formula that leads to sustained weight loss today.

As obesity became more prevalent throughout the eighteenth century, so too did accounts of personal struggles with weight, along with the inevitable revolutionary prescription for recovery. These prescriptions varied dramatically in their details, but they always agreed that fatty meats made you fat. The English physician George Cheyne described obesity as a new "English Malady," known "only to the Rich, the Lazy, the Luxurious," who are "furnished with the rarest Delicacies, the richest Foods, and the most generous Wines." He himself was afflicted, and only succeeded in recovering with a strict diet of "seeds, bread, mealy roots, and fruit," along with milk and vegetables. Similar cases abound in the medical literature of the time, and they all laid blame on fatty meats and high-fat dairy products.

For all of these physicians, an Atkins-style diet allowing near limitless consumption of meat and dairy fat would have seemed preposterous. In his authoritative and widely reprinted 1813 *Cursory Remarks on Corpulence; or Obesity Considered as a Disease*, William Wadd describes how the majority of his patients, and his largest patients, were "persons indulging in fat animal food." When people eliminated animal food, he observed, they often lost weight, providing "strong evidence of the efficacy of vegetable diet." Most of the authorities he cites also recommend a vegetarian diet, accompanied, perhaps, by a small quantity of lean meat.

But unlike those who came before him, Wadd acknowledged that ultimately, the *type* of food you consume is a secondary issue. He had to, because the formula of *you are what you eat* didn't fit with the evidence available to him. His book recounts numerous cases of people becoming fat without consuming any meat: the "rich and opulent" in Italy whose "chief food consists of vegetable production"; Chinese slaves in the sugar season who get fat "without any other sustenance than the ripe sugar cane." There was no denying that vegetarians gained weight despite avoiding animal products.

After carefully evaluating the evidence, Wadd parted company with previous diet gurus by refusing to favor one type of food over another as a means of losing weight. "Of the efficacy of animal or vegetable food in the reduction of corpulency, there can be no just preference given to either," he concluded, "*quantity,* and not *quality,* being the only point to be attended to."

That should have been that. *You are what you eat* isn't true; *you are how much you eat* is the real equation. No just preference can be given to low fat *or* low carb. Quantity is the issue. Wadd's voice was the voice of common sense, and his conclusion is the only one supported by current science. So why did people continue to demonize fatty meat?

Virtuous Vegetarians and Cruel Carnivores

Wadd's book appeared at a key moment in the history of food, coincident with the beginnings of modern vegetarianism. The diagnosis of obesity as a disease of modernity had gained widespread acceptance. Disgusted with their sinful society and its attendant sicknesses, people sought answers, as they always do, in mythic visions of paradise past, when humans lived innocently and free of all physical ailments. The pernicious effects of fatty meat were elegantly explained by our tragic departure from the natural and virtuous vegetarian habits of a better time.

For nineteenth-century vegetarians, obesity was only the latest and gravest punishment for our consumption of the wrong foods, meat chief among them. Their version of paradise past—in which we only ate vegetables—gained strength from the logic of *you are what you eat.* Eating *badly*—that is, immorally—will make you feel bad. Following this logic, in 1813 the vegetarian poet Percy Bysshe Shelley penned *A Vindication of Natural Diet*, in which he held that physical and moral failings in man were due to unnatural and vicious dietary habits. "Man," Shelley argued, "and the animals whom he has infected with his society [are] alone diseased." In his fantasy world, wild hogs, bison, and wolves died only of external violence or old age, but domestic hogs, sheep, cows, and dogs suffered from "an incredible variety of distempers; and, like the corrupters of their nature, have physicians who thrive upon their miseries." Man the meat eater was a "pimp for the gluttony of death." We should emulate the first Christians, Shelley wrote, who lived long because they practiced abstinence from animal flesh.

Two years after the publication of *A Vindication of Natural Diet*, a doctor and close friend of Shelley's named William Lambe used the supposed connection between obesity and animal fat to generalize about the dangers of eating meat. In his book *Water and Vegetable Diet in Consumption, Scrofula, Cancer, Asthma, and Other Chronic Diseases*, Lambe recounted the famous case of a miller named Thomas Wood, who had become exceedingly fat on a diet of strong ale, "animal food," and "large quantities of butter and cheese." Wood recovered on a vegetarian diet of sea biscuits and flour pudding made with skim milk or water—proof, for Lambe, that a vegetable regimen made you live longer. "It affords no trifling grounds of suspicion against animal food," warned Lambe, "that it so obviously inclines to corpulency." Vegetarianism wasn't just virtuous—it cured cancer and asthma and melted off the pounds.

Among the vegetarians influenced by Lambe and Shelley, the most influential was probably Sylvester Graham, inventor of the graham cracker and the Graham diet. In the 1830s, Graham touted his vegetarian dietary regimen as a cure for everything from chronic disease to violent tendencies and excessive sexual desire: just as eating fat makes you fat, eating animals exacerbates your animal instincts, in turn increasing your appetite for food and sex. To support his claims, Graham dutifully collected anecdotes of vegetarian longevity and perfect health. And to justify his arguments against eating meat, he appealed to evolutionary biology—"man is not provided with sharpness of fangs." Yet the real strength of his message lay not in science or empirical evidence, but rather in the persuasive power of sympathetic magical thinking— and like today, people were willing to believe in magic.

Changing Diets, Unchanging Myths

The rule that dieters should avoid fatty meat remained more or less constant in late-nineteenth- and early-twentieth-century America. California citrus producers popularized the Hollywood Eighteen-Day Diet, consisting of grapefruit, toast, black coffee, and raw vegetables for dinner. Dieters who prioritized simplicity could choose from a variety of popular two-food diets: coffee and doughnuts, baked potatoes and buttermilk, raw tomatoes and hard-boiled eggs, and, of course, the bananas and skim milk once used by Dr. Sidney Haas to treat celiac. There was the grapefruit juice diet, the "slo-baked" Wonder Bread that helped you "diet with a smile," and Welch's grape juice that "burned up ugly fat." Americans obsessed with slimness were willing to believe almost any absurdity—yet only one popular diet allowed for fatty meat. This was the pineapple and lamb chop diet—and only because the acidic pineapple would "digest" the lamb, neutralizing its ability to make you fat. (It was a smash hit at the University of Michigan and Smith College in the 1920s.)

Without taking into account the long tradition of connecting fatty meat, obesity, and poor health, we cannot fully understand the core myth that underwrites Harvard's continued prohibition of butter and Americans' fear of fat. When Taubes describes this core myth as the "changing-American-diet story," he is only partially right:

> The changing-American-diet story envisions the turn of the century as an idyllic era free of chronic disease, and then portrays Americans as brought low by the inexorable spread of fat and meat into the American diet. It has been repeated so often that it has taken on the semblance of indisputable truth—but this conclusion is based on remarkably insubstantial and contradictory evidence.

It's true that this story formed an important part of the most recent crusade against dietary fat, led by researchers like Ancel Keys. But Keys did not come up with the story. Like so many before him, when it came to eating fatty meat he simply clothed the powerful formula of *you are what you eat* in flashy new science. Doctors like Dean Ornish and Caldwell Esselstyn who praise vegetarian diets as the best way to lose weight and get healthy should listen to William Wadd. *There can be no just preference given to vegetable food.* Studies that "prove" otherwise are nothing more than the latest rationalization of an empirically unverified myth: eating fat, particularly fatty meat, makes you fat and sick.

Don't think for a moment that science makes us immune to magical thinking. Modern educated Americans may not eat tiger meat to increase their strength, but *you are what you eat* still plays a significant role in our intuitions about the effects of certain foods—even

Don't think for a moment that science makes us immune to magical thinking.

when we aren't aware of it. To demonstrate the subconscious influence of this myth on American college students, psychologist Paul Rozin devised an ingenious test. He and his associates wrote two descriptions of a tribal society called the "Chandorans," which included information about hunting, diet, and family. The descriptions were identical in nearly every respect, down to what the Chandorans hunted: boar and marine turtle. But in one description, the Chandorans hunt marine turtle exclusively for its shell, and eat only boar. In the other description, the Chandorans hunt boar exclusively for its tusks, and eat only marine turtle.

When asked to rate the Chandorans in categories such as longevity and speed, students significantly associated consumption of turtle with longevity and slowness. Conversely, consumption of boar was associated with being heavyset and aggressive. The results, stated Rozin, "are clearly consistent with the hypothesis that, at some level, subjects 'believe' that 'you are what you eat.'"

In another study, psychologist Michael Oakes examined whether fat content or calorie content was more important for people judging a food's perceived capacity to promote weight gain. To his great surprise, Oakes discovered that a single Snickers miniature—47 calories—was perceived to promote more weight gain than a *569-calorie buffet of cottage cheese, carrots, and pears*. Not only that, the erroneous perception was mediated almost entirely by fat content. High sugar content did not produce the same effect. "The weight-enhancing effects of foods," reported Oakes, "appear to revolve around fat content more so than any other characteristic of foods (including amounts of calories)."

The term for this phenomenon is "health halo," coined in 2006 by marketing professors Pierre Chandon and Brian Wansink, the latter of whom is director of Cornell's Food and Brand Lab and the author of *Mindless Eating* and *Slim by Design*. To test the effects of low-fat labels on food consumption, Wansink and Chandon put out two bowls of gold, teal, purple, and white M&M's. Each bowl had a professionally designed label—one read "New Colors of Regular M&M's," the other read "New 'Low-Fat' M&M's." Participants in the study who served themselves from the low-fat bowl ate 28.4 percent more M&M's, a figure that rose to 47 percent among the study's overweight participants. "Health halos," suggested the researchers, "lead consumers to believe that the food contains fewer calories and that the acceptable or appropriate amount to consume is higher when the food is described as being lower in fat." Given the historical influence of *you are what you eat*, it's likely that 200 years ago their study would have yielded similar results.

The Dangers of Fat Magic

We may not know which diet is best for losing weight, but one thing is clear: failure to recognize the power of magical thinking in dietary science has negative real-world consequences. Seductive myths continue to inspire irrational fear of fat—in scientists, in governments, and in the general public. The result is a cacophony of conflicting dietary advice, none of which actually helps us get healthier, an unpleasant truth borne out by the persistent failure of this advice to effect change in the public's eating habits.

These myths also underwrite less obvious instances of irrationality, often with devastating consequences. Take commonsense understandings of obesity. Even among those who reject the idea that eating fat makes you fat, the cause of obesity is usually conceptualized as some combination of failed self-control and poor nutritional choices. *You are what you eat* puts the emphasis on *you* (failed self-control) and what *you* choose to eat.

Does that really make sense? UCLA sociologist Abigail Saguy has made the case that it doesn't. To highlight the irrationality of attributing obesity to personal responsibility, Saguy compared media treatments of obesity and anorexia. Unsurprisingly, she found that a "personal responsibility frame" dominated coverage of obesity. Fat people, explains Saguy, are predominantly depicted as lazy and/or ignorant. She quotes a characteristic op-ed by George F. Will, "Sex, Fat, and Responsibility," in which Will asserts that "Americans are becoming fatter because they are becoming more slothful and self-indulgent." There is something wrong with *you*.

Saguy emphasizes that medical professionals are similarly biased. In a study of 620 primary care physicians in the United States, one-third felt their obese patients were "weak-willed, sloppy, and lazy," and more than 50 percent characterized them as "awkward, unattractive, ugly, or noncompliant." Like George Will and everyone else who blames fat people for being fat, physicians have been hypnotized by the *you* in *you are what you eat*. If you are eating too much, then the fault must lie in *you*.

The same does not hold for anorexia, Saguy notes. Since anorexics are defined by what they don't eat, *you are what you eat* no longer applies, and in media treatments of anorexia, environmental and genetic factors take precedence over narratives of personal responsibility. Anorexics are rarely derided as weak-willed followers of unrealistic body image standards. No one would ever say, "Just start eating, you lazy weakling!" to an anorexic. When someone isn't eating, there is no *you* to blame. ("No one to blame" is the subtitle of a 2005 *Newsweek* article about anorexia.) The opposite is true of the obese, who are portrayed as weakly submitting to gluttonous impulses. And the result is unwarranted blame and shame—even among the medical professionals we trust to be free from the influence of magical thinking.

It's not just a myopic focus on *you* that can be problematic. In the quest to understand obesity, the myth of *you are what you eat* results in endless studies and debates about what's wrong with what we *eat*. Yet an increasingly vocal minority of researchers are rejecting this emphasis, led by biostatistician and professor of public health David B. Allison. In 2011, Allison and coauthors published the results of research on animal populations living with or around humans in industrialized societies—lab animals, domestic pets, and feral rats. The study, titled "Canaries in the coal mine: a cross-species analysis of the plurality of obesity epidemics," showed that the body weight of all animal populations had risen over the last three decades. This result was particularly unexpected in the case of lab animals, whose diets and living conditions remained nearly constant. Animals were managing to get fatter, "even in the absence of those factors that are typically conceived of as the primary determinants of the human obesity epidemic via their influence on diet (e.g., access to vending machines)."

Without questioning the relevance of diet to weight gain, Allison and others are calling for obesity researchers to abandon an exclusive *you are what you eat* model of what makes us fat. They cite a number of understudied possible contributors, all of which are supported by empirical evidence and prior plausibility. Among these are increased sleep debt, reduction in variability of ambient temperature (air conditioners and heaters), decreased smoking, mood stabilizers, chronic stress, higher average maternal age, and obesogens—chemical compounds commonly used in the manufacture of food containers that may be disrupting lipid metabolism.

The lesson to be learned from all this is not that eating saturated fat doesn't make you fat, or that willpower has no relationship to weight loss. Rather, it's that determining and properly weighting the effects of diet on health is tremendously difficult. Too often, "established facts" like the dangers of saturated fat are not facts at all, but intuitively plausible conjectures that attract disproportionate amounts of attention and research. And their plausibility, in large part, comes from an unacknowledged appeal to myths and magical thinking.

Public health advocates must learn to be humble about what they know and careful with what they say. If trotting out one set of dietary recommendations after another has no discernible effect on Americans other than to make them paranoid and irrational, why issue recommendations unless we are *absolutely sure* they make sense? Nobody thinks that a moderate diet high in saturated fat is the primary cause of obesity and heart disease in America. And we already have a basic goal everyone can agree on: getting people to eat less food and be more active. Advocates should focus their efforts on that, before moving on to hash out the controversial details of proper food ratios and ideal forms of exercise. When they don't, their authority suffers. Since rules about the right amount of fat aren't based on sound science, they vary from one source to the next. The AHA advocates keeping total dietary fat *of any kind* to between 25 and 35 percent of daily calories. Meanwhile, the Harvard School of Public Health states that there is no "maximum on the percentage of calories people should get each day from healthy sources of fat . . . the opposite of the low-fat message promoted for decades by the USDA." This kind of conflict opens the door to anti-establishment diet gurus who exploit the seeming inconsistency of mainstream authorities to promote their own crackpot theories. Better, instead, to present a united front, at least until the basic goal of getting people to eat in moderation has been achieved. To insist on issuing highly specific nutritional guidelines is manifestly not in the public interest; it is in the interest of those who, from the time of Galen onward, have made scientific and political careers out of issuing guidelines more complicated than simply eating in moderation.

So next time you feel guilty about eating butter or crispy chicken skin, try to remember the source of that guilt. Remember the tiger penises. Remember Galen and his snails. But don't be disappointed if all that remembering doesn't completely overcome the force of myth. After all, it hasn't for Steven Shapin, a Harvard historian of science who specializes in the history of dietetics and has written extensively on the history of *you are what you eat.*

"Academically, I understand the history of these rules, their uncertainty," Shapin tells me in a phone interview. "I teach my students to be aware of the history. But in the real world I think Hume is right. The philosopher's skepticism vanishes like smoke outside of his study."

He pauses for a moment, and when he speaks I can almost hear a rueful smile.

"That's why in my fridge there's still a tub of I Can't Believe It's Not Butter."

CHAPTER FOUR

Sugar Crazy

Let's Blame Sugar Instead!

It seems we can't live without nutritional wars. Yes, medical professionals have admitted they exaggerated the dangers of saturated fat. And yes, *Time* magazine ran a June 2014 cover story called "Ending the War on Fat." But that doesn't mean you can relax—far from it. Not two months later, *Time* ran another article: "How Sweet Can Become Toxic."

For many health-conscious Americans, the article confirmed common knowledge: the war on sugar had already begun. Take a look at some of the terrifying headlines from the past couple of years:

"SUGARY BEVERAGES LINKED TO
180,000 DEATHS WORLDWIDE"
—*Time.com, March 2013*

"Sugar Is Killing Us, and It Doesn't Take Much"
—*Salon.com, February 2014*

"Sweet Poison: How sugar, not cocaine, is one
of the most addictive and dangerous substances"
—New York Daily News, *February 10, 2014*

The 2014 documentary *Fed Up,* narrated by television journalist Katie Couric, featured a slew of experts calling sugar toxic, poisonous, and evil. The filmmakers provide a litany of sobering statistics on the documentary's website:

- In 2012, Americans consumed an average of 765 grams of sugar every five days, or 130 pounds each year.

- One soda a day increases a child's chance of obesity by 60 percent.

- Individuals who drink one to two sugar-sweetened beverages per day have a 26 percent higher risk for developing type 2 diabetes.

The website encouraged visitors to sign up for a detoxifying ten-day sugar-free "challenge," developed in close consultation with Dr. Mark Hyman, a frequent guest on *The Dr. Oz Show*, personal doctor to the Clintons, and author of *The Blood Sugar Solution 10-Day Detox Diet: Activate Your Body's Natural Ability to Burn Fat and Lose Weight Fast.*

Participants in the detox challenge received daily e-mails that summarized recent revelations about sugar. One warned of sugar's many disguises—it has fifty-six names! (For you religion buffs, that's fifteen more than Satan.) Like some secular version of kosher law, the challenge called on people to scour their kitchens and rid them of any items with added sugar, including jams and jellies, soy sauce, ketchup, and even fruit juices with only naturally occurring sugar. A representative tip: "Sugar by any name still does your body harm!"

Addictive! Poisonous! Dangerous! Deadly! It may sound like hyperbole, but all these media sources cite scientific studies and medical professionals who assure us that this time we have identified a genuine supervillain. Promise. At the beginning of 2014, the World Health Organization reviewed the science and issued its new guidelines on sugar consumption: ideally no more than 5 percent of your daily calories should come from added sugar. In a 2,000-calorie diet, that's 100 calories. A 12-ounce Coke has 140 calories, which means just one soda puts you over the WHO's recommendation. For coffee and tea drinkers, teaspoons might be a more helpful measurement: the WHO allows six per day.

But here's the thing: if sugar is an addictive toxin, then the WHO doesn't go far enough. It's not merely people stirring Cokes with Twizzlers who need to scale back sugar consumption. Nor is scaling back a reasonable approach. Sugar, we are told, is like cigarettes and cocaine—and there is no "safe" level of cocaine or tobacco consumption. You wouldn't give your children bourbon and cigarettes on their birthday, so it's probably wise not to feed them that toxic slice of cake. And you wouldn't let them have just one puff from a cigarette every day, which is what the WHO seems to allow. We need to rethink *everything* about our culinary culture in light of these shocking new scientific developments.

Sugar, we are told, is like cigarettes and cocaine—and there is no "safe" level of cocaine or tobacco consumption.

Is Alice Waters the Devil?

In fact, if sugar is evil, even celebrity chef and food activist Alice Waters, a pioneer of local, organic farming, could be a villain in disguise.

One of Waters's many accomplishments is a program called Edible Schoolyard (ESY), which encourages urban public middle schoolers to grow and harvest their own produce in an organic garden, then cook it themselves in a kitchen classroom.

Waters sees ESY as a first step in the fight against what she calls the "insidious," "dishonest" culture of fast food.

"We're in the middle of a health epidemic," says Waters. "If we could somehow bring in a curriculum around school lunch, we could change the way kids think about eating."

But what about the fact that "sugar is killing us, and it doesn't take much"? If sugar alarmists are to be believed, teachers at the Edible Schoolyard in Berkeley, California, are also encouraging students to become addicts. Apparently Waters never warned curriculum supervisors about the most potent unregulated culinary toxin on the market. The opening paragraph of a 2004 ESY profile reads like Big Sugar propaganda: "The apple crisp is baking in the oven and the smell of bubbling cinnamon, sugar, and apples fills the air and makes the kitchen feel warm and cozy." The Edible Schoolyard website even features a recipe for "Celebratory Apple Crisp."

What are they celebrating? Type 2 diabetes? The obesity epidemic? The worst addiction facing today's youth? Just one serving of a typical crisp recipe packs a whopping 11 teaspoons of sugar, which is almost *twice* the maximum daily amount allowed for children by the WHO. And forget about throwing vanilla ice cream on there, homemade or otherwise—that's another 5 teaspoons of sugar. Might as well teach those kids how to freebase crack on an actual teaspoon.

Fortunately, Alice Waters is not a villain. Science has *not* shown that sugar is addictive. The statistics cited in *Fed Up* and the alarmist headlines misrepresent research and needlessly frighten the public. The newly declared war on sugar, like the war on fat, is the misguided work of overconfident scientists and a media that thrives on fear. Don't fall for it. After you see the history and listen to the experts who aren't as obsessed with publicity, you'll want to bake a delicious dessert and celebrate your freedom from a culture of food paranoia.

Big Sugar's Sweet Lies

The current crusade against sugar can be traced to the work of one vociferous expert, Dr. Robert Lustig, an endocrinologist and childhood obesity specialist at the prestigious University of California, San Francisco School of Medicine.

Lustig's rise to stardom began in 2009, when his PowerPoint presentation, "Sugar: The Bitter Truth," went viral on YouTube. In the video, Lustig pronounces the scientific evidence decisive. Sugar is "evil," "toxic," "poisonous," and "addictive." Armed with an arsenal of citations and authoritative lessons on metabolic function, he asserts that sugar, not an excess of calories, is the primary factor in obesity, in part because it is addictive. Tobacco, alcohol, cocaine, heroin, and morphine feature as prominent analogies throughout his follow-up best-selling book, *Fat Chance*. (There is no recipe for "Celebratory Apple Crisp" in *The Fat Chance Cookbook*, though there are a few low-sugar dessert recipes at the end, like an obligatory dance for guests at a Puritan wedding: "This [apple] pie is as 'safe' as you can make a pie." Enjoy!)

Lustig's arguments, and his apocalyptic rhetoric, have won over prominent policy makers and journalists. Among them is science writer Gary Taubes, the same skeptic who made his name undermining exaggerated claims about the dangers of saturated fat. In 2011, Taubes wrote an article for the *New York Times* titled "Is Sugar Toxic?," a rhetorical question he answered in the affirmative. Lustig is "persuasive," concludes Taubes. Not only is sugar "the primary reason that the numbers of obese and diabetic Americans have skyrocketed in the past 30 years," but sugar "is also the likely dietary cause of several other chronic ailments widely considered to be diseases of Western lifestyles—heart disease, hypertension, and many common cancers among them." That a skeptic like Taubes could be convinced of sugar's toxicity lent credibility to the notion that science had finally discovered the dietary equivalent of Hitler—pure, white, and deadly.

Sugar itself isn't the only problem: we are told that the people who produce and sell it are evil, too. Lustig and others point out how sugar benefits from a heavy-hitting propaganda machine, in the form of corporate lobbyists and scientists from Big Sugar and Big Food. These corrupt corporate interests, they argue, have kept us from the horrific truth about their products.

The evidence on this score is damning. A 2013 systematic review, for instance, examined studies about the correlation between sugar-sweetened beverages and obesity, paying close attention to financial conflicts of interest with corporations and special interest groups such as Coca-Cola, Pepsi, the Corn Refiners Association, the Sugar Association, Archer Daniels Midland, Cargill, and British sugar giant Tate & Lyle. When financial conflicts of interest were present, there was an 83 percent chance the study would show no correlation between sugar-sweetened beverage consumption and obesity. Studies without a financial conflict of interest, on the other hand, overwhelmingly supported an association. Clearly industry funding skewed results in favor of sugar.

These conflicts of interest often hide from the public behind academic journal paywalls, and are sometimes undisclosed entirely. In a 2014 exposé, the *Washington Post* reported on how the Corn Refiners Association gave Harvard-trained cardiologist and Tufts University professor James Rippe more than $10 million in research funds, as well as a $41,000 monthly retainer to serve as an expert consultant. The results of Rippe's research, unsurprisingly, exonerate high-fructose corn syrup. Yet Rippe managed to become the editor of Springer Books' 2014 reference book, *Fructose, High Fructose Corn Syrup, Sucrose, and Health*. The online "about the author" section catalogs Dr. Rippe's extensive credentials and professional accomplishments—but his connections to the Corn Refiners Association are nowhere to be found.

The same groups funding studies and paying consulting fees have also been working furiously to influence politics. In *Mother Jones* magazine, Taubes and coauthor Cristin Kearns Couzens documented how Big Sugar "used Big Tobacco–style tactics to ensure that government agencies would dismiss troubling health claims against their products," starting in the 1970s. They cite Lustig's research that "sucrose and high-fructose corn syrup are addictive in much the same way as cigarettes and alcohol." Why doesn't the public know these startling facts, ask the authors? Because the Sugar Association continues to use illegitimate studies by paid researchers like James Rippe to assert that Lustig's evidence against sugar is inconclusive. Then they pay lobbyists to poison politicians with that corrupt science.

In light of this unconscionable corporate manipulation, the recent backlash against Big Sugar seems like a victory of truth over deception. The story is appealingly simple: sugar, and its producers, are evil, and they are responsible for the world's rising rates of obesity, type 2 diabetes, and other chronic diseases. Consumers are caught in the middle of an epic struggle. Our expanding waistlines aren't due to lack of willpower, because sugar is addictive. Best of all, the solution to this simple problem is equally simple: regulate sugar like the dangerous drug that it is.

Or is it?

The Bitter Truth: Science Is Complicated

Evil corporations poisoning innocent children. Corrupt Big Sugar against virtuous scientists. These black-and-white pairings make for great stories with high outrage appeal. But uncomplicated tales of good and evil belong in myths and fairy tales, not science. When I contacted endocrinologists who specialized in diabetes, they consistently refused to confirm the idea of sugar as a toxic villain. One referred to Lustig by name as extreme and opinionated. Others made it clear that the science on sugar is far from settled, and extremism at this time is irresponsible. Speaking with them reinforced an important fact: *just because Big Sugar says the science isn't settled doesn't automatically prove the opposite.*

Confronted with genuinely bad science that attacks a product—anti-vaccine activism, for instance—industries will naturally weigh in on the debate and pay scientists to evaluate the truth of the accusations against them. When Taubes was busy debunking alarmism about saturated fat, the dairy and beef industries were busy sponsoring studies and lobbying politicians to tone down the anti-fat rhetoric. (They still do.) That means Taubes was aligning himself *with* industry, which made it hard for him to get heard. At the time, any suggestion that saturated fat might not be *so* bad was discredited through association with corporate interests. That turned out to be a mistake. Could the same thing be happening with sugar? Are we allowing hatred of Big Food to get in the way of good science?

I have talked extensively about this possibility with Dr. Philip Zeitler, the head of endocrinology at Children's Hospital Colorado and one of the world's leading experts on type 2 diabetes in children. Zeitler is no sugar industry stooge. He has no conflicts of interest to disclose: no viral YouTube video, no celebrity patients, and no bestselling book—just patients and peer-reviewed journal articles. He speaks passionately about his work helping children lose weight, avoid type 2 diabetes, and eat more healthfully. He also speaks passionately against sensationalist anti-sugar rhetoric.

"Unfortunately there are plenty of researchers that are happy to become excitable for the media," he says. "Certain people believe that fructose is particularly poisonous. I think the evidence for that is interesting, but not nearly as convincing as some loud people would suggest."

Zeitler runs through various theories about why sugar, and fructose particularly, might be especially bad for our health and waistlines. But, like gluten researcher Peter Gibson, he emphasizes that responsible scientists shouldn't jump to conclusions.

"People are coming to the data with substantial biases," Zeitler says. "Fructose is not a smoking gun. And there's been too much gunjumping around food, which is something that people take incredibly seriously. That's a disservice to the public, to science, and to people's understanding of how science works. People want to hear about something simple and magical, not a complex situation. Diabetes is incredibly complex. Most of what we know now has been discovered in the last five years, and we don't know very much."

So when it comes to diabetes, fructose isn't a smoking gun. But what about the theory that sugar is addictive? Lustig devotes an entire chapter of *Fat Chance* to the topic: "Food Addiction—Fact or Fallacy." His answer is clear. "Although the brain's reward system is complex," Lustig writes, "it can be reduced to the 'hedonic pathway.'" Sugar stimulates this pathway, just like "drugs of abuse such as nicotine, cocaine, morphine, and alcohol." Readers are instructed to think about soda as a "fructose delivery vehicle, similar to cigarettes."

Experts on addiction disagree. Contra Lustig's oversimplified chapter title, there's a giant gray area of uncertainty between scientific "facts" and "fallacies," and that's where theories of food addiction, including sugar addiction, currently belong. Among the skeptics are two Cambridge scholars, psychiatrist and eating behavior specialist Hisham Ziauddeen and neuroscientist Paul Fletcher, both of whom think the food addiction model has serious shortcomings.

"Addiction literature is not nearly as straightforward as it is made out to be," Ziauddeen explains to me. "One difficulty is that our entire conceptualization of addiction was originally built around substances you don't need to take. Once you start talking about food addiction, it's hard to know what addiction means. Can you be addicted to skiing? Sex? There are no clear-cut answers to these questions, and no agreed-upon ways to test them."

I ask Ziauddeen about the media's focus on studies that show how eating sugar lights up parts of the brain associated with drug use.

"You can show the brain any reward— sugar, alcohol, sex, a movie— and it will light up. That says nothing about things being addictive."

"That technology and its capabilities have been communicated incorrectly," says Ziauddeen, clearly exasperated. "You can show the brain any reward— sugar, alcohol, sex, a movie—and it will light up. That says nothing about things being addictive, even though it's pre-sented that way. All it demonstrates is that the brain is doing what it is sup-posed to do. In neuroimaging there is no clear-cut sign of addiction."

It is simply false to assert that sugar's role in diabetes, addiction, and obesity has been settled. A late 2013 state-of-the-field piece in the journal *Metabolism* by three Harvard en-docrinologists examined the evidence to date about the health effects of sugar. Their conclusion? "Much more research is [. . .] needed."

Now that's real science.

If It Tastes Good It Must Be Bad

If the science isn't settled, why are people—and policy-making orga-nizations like the WHO—so willing to condemn sugar? Long before Lustig and *Fed Up*, psychologist Paul Rozin set out to answer this ques-tion in his 1987 essay, "Sweetness, Sensuality, Sin, Safety, and Socializa-tion: Some Speculations." In it, Rozin hypothesized that for Americans, fear of sugar is a manifestation of subconscious Puritan values, the be-lief that "anything that is extremely pleasurable, and that includes sex

and sweetness, must be bad." Two decades later, Rozin believes very little has changed, and a form of secular puritanism continues to inform
our food taboos. Rigorous science has nothing to do with it.

"Like religion, people's attitude toward food is very evidence insensitive," he tells me. "And then science can go on a jag and get religious
on something, especially in Protestant countries like the US." Regarding our attitude toward sugar, Rozin recounts an experiment he performed in which people from America and France were asked to word
associate with "chocolate cake."

"The Americans chose 'guilt' and the French chose 'celebration,'"
Rozin says. "There's a serious difference between our food cultures,
which we've shown again and again, and it doesn't come down to scientific evidence that we've got and they don't."

One important factor in sugar extremism is something Rozin calls
"the monotonic mind." A person who thinks monotonically has difficulty accepting that low and high doses of a particular substance
may have opposite effects. This type of thinking is associated with religious categorizations of foods as pure or impure, moral or immoral.
For an Orthodox Jew, a tiny bite of bacon and a pork chop are both
forbidden—pork's impurity is *monotonic*.

But nutrition isn't monotonic. A glass of wine a day won't kill you,
and theories that it's good for you go in and out of fashion. Yet forty
glasses of wine will definitely kill you: low and high doses can have opposite effects. This phenomenon, known as dose-sensitivity, is a basic
tenet of toxicology, put most famously by Renaissance scientist Para-
celsus: "The dose makes the poison." While this isn't universally true—
exposure to HIV is monotonic—it certainly holds for sugar.

Despite the obvious dose-sensitivity of food, evidence suggests that
large numbers of people think monotonically about sugar. In a 1996
survey, nearly a third of Americans agreed that a diet free of sugar was
healthier than a diet with just a pinch of sugar in it. This irrational

monotonic bias is puzzling, unless you combine two beliefs: (1) Sugar is deadly in moderate doses, and (2) it is addictive. These, of course, are beliefs that hold for drugs of abuse. Even if one line of cocaine won't kill you, the risk of addiction means that even a little cocaine is potentially very dangerous. Thus, if sugar is addictive, it makes sense to treat it monotonically—a little could easily become a lot, and a lot could have devastating consequences.

It turns out that in 1996 the public already had good reason to view sugar as a deadly drug. Food historian Harvey Levenstein describes how the '60s and '70s saw an explosion of "sucrophobia" in Britain and America. At the time, Ancel Keys was busy defaming saturated fat, to the great consternation of American dairy, meat, and egg producers. But on the other side of the Atlantic, British scientist John Yudkin had developed a different theory. According to Yudkin, Keys had it all wrong. Sugar, not saturated fat, was the real dietary villain.

Yudkin experimented on rats, feeding some sugar and others starch and saturated fat. The sugar-fed ones were a mess: higher cholesterol, higher blood pressure, higher fasting glucose levels, and much fatter than their starch-and-fat-fed counterparts. These dramatic results confirmed what Yudkin found when analyzing the health of various populations according to their sugar intake. His powerful argument received a great deal of press in England, and in 1972 he wrote a widely read book titled *Pure, Sweet, and Dangerous: The New Facts about the Sugar You Eat as a Cause of Heart Disease, Diabetes, and Other Killers.* Delighted by this alternative theory, the National Commission on Egg Nutrition in America (industry science!) invited Yudkin on a media tour, during which he counseled people to eat less sugar and continue to eat eggs, much to the dismay of the American Heart Association. (Yudkin's book was republished by Penguin in 2012 as *Pure, White and Deadly*, with a preface by Lustig, who refers to Yudkin as a "prophet" and himself as a "disciple" and an "acolyte.")

While Yudkin was somewhat circumspect about sugar's addictiveness—he called himself a sugar "addict" in scare quotes, and said it was "weakly" addictive—contemporaries were not. In 1968, the influential food activist Jerome Irving Rodale wrote *Natural Health, Sugar, and the Criminal Mind*, in which he blamed sugar for everything from rape to the rise of Nazism. (Three years later, Rodale went on *The Dick Cavett Show* and said he'd decided to "live to be a hundred," just before dropping dead of a heart attack onstage. His company, Rodale Inc., lives on, and among its many, many best sellers is *Wheat Belly*. It is also responsible for *The Biggest Loser*.) And in 1975, American nutritionist William Dufty published *Sugar Blues*, a best seller that described sugar addiction as "the white plague," food products as "laced with sugar," and his own habit as "the road to perdition."

Not only were adults like Dufty succumbing to addiction, but children were eating sugar and going crazy. A year before *Sugar Blues* came out, the American Academy of Pediatrics published a letter to the editor from a Dr. William Crook that originated the connection between sugar and hyperactivity in children. "Only within the past three years," wrote Crook, "have I become aware that sugar . . . more especially cane sugar . . . is a leading cause of hyperactivity." Just like MSG sensitivity—which also started with a letter—the myth of sugar hyperactivity *still* commands popular belief, despite having been thoroughly debunked. Again and again researchers have failed to demonstrate that children who eat sugar become hyperactive, as documented by the National Institute of Mental Health, but parents still live in fear. (Old Navy sells a "Let's Blame the Sugar" T-shirt for babies.) Once a dietary myth has been introduced, it's very, very hard to eradicate.

It would be one thing if all this concern about sugar were the result of legitimate scientific inquiry, which always produces a few false alarms. But the demonization of sugar goes back far further than John

Yudkin's hapless rats. Sugar was labeled addictive and toxic before brain scans and the childhood obesity epidemic, before concerns about type 2 diabetes, before Lustig's paradisiacal 1960s, when "soda was a treat and available only in 12-ounce cans."

Rozin's hypothesis is entirely accurate. The reasons for sucrophobia have always had little to do with science, and everything to do with moralism, superstition, and puritanical fear of sinful pleasures. This is just another case of myth disguised as science, and after you travel back a few hundred years and see the roots of the myth for yourself, I think you'll be as fed up as I am.

The Sugar Invasion

Granular sucrose, the result of processing liquid from sugarcane grass, remained a rarity in Europe until the sixteenth century. First introduced from the Middle East during the Crusades, sugar was for centuries considered a spice and a medicine, consumed, as the thirteenth-century church father Thomas Aquinas wrote, not "with the end in mind of nourishment, but rather for ease of digestion."

According to sugar historian Sidney Mintz, European use of sugar as a "condiment" really took off in the seventeenth century, due to the rising popularity of three new "bitter stimulant" beverages: coffee, tea, and chocolate. Mintz traces the earliest medical concern about sugar to this same period, starting with the 1633 publication of *The Diet of the Diseased*, by Puritan British physician James Hart. Hart, a traditionalist, disapproved of how foreign "sugar hath now succeeded hon[ey]." He confirmed anecdotal observations—now well established as scientific fact—that "immoderate" consumption of sugar "rots the teeth, making them look black, and, withal, causes many times a loathsome stinking breath." That much was true—but because of his bias in favor of honey, Hart neglected to mention, or perhaps never noticed, that it, too, can rot the teeth.

It was only a matter of time before baseless, speculative dangers joined cavities on the list of ills associated with processed sugar. At first, these speculations were born of sugar's association with tea and coffee, which traditionalists saw as exotic, unnatural fads. Eighteenth-century reformer Jonas Hanway described tea as the "cause of many distempers." According to Hanway, this new beverage was liable to create "fantastic desires and bad habits in which nature has no part," aided by an equally "pernicious Foreigner, called *Sugar*." Children, Hanway warned, were particularly susceptible to sugar's detrimental effects, which included "scurvy [and] weak nerves."

Sugar was a strange, modern food, and it fit the ever-recurring myth of modernity as evil and the past as good. This new foreign invader made a perfect scapegoat to blame for the intractable illnesses of the time. Instead of obesity and diabetes, the eighteenth-century public was worried about scurvy, weak nerves, and sexuality ("bad habits in which nature has no part"). There was, of course, no evidence that sugar produced scurvy, just as there was no evidence that tea could create "fantastic desires." But it didn't matter—the argument against sugar drew on its origin, not empirical evidence.

Sugar also seemed unhealthy because of a different kind of origin: immoral production methods. Religious food taboos have long maintained that if you eat something with a *morally* bad origin—unblessed meat, for example—then there will be *physically* bad consequences. We saw this superstition at work when vegetarians who opposed the slaughter of animals on moral grounds converted that immoral origin into the perceived health dangers of meat. When Hart and Hanway were writing, British sugar consumers had to reckon with a different kind of evil origin: slavery. At the time, sugar was the fruit of slave labor in the West Indies. Abolitionists called on all Christians to boycott "products defiled with blood." Anti-sugar advocates urged adults to drink unsweetened coffee and tea, and children were asked to forgo sweets to prevent "the selling of their little black brothers into bondage."

Sugar is no longer produced by slaves, but modern anti-sugar advocates continue to invoke its immoral origins. In Michael Moss's *Salt Sugar Fat: How the Food Giants Hooked Us*, Big Food's soullessness is front and center. Following in the footsteps of Hanway and Hart, the first section on sugar is titled "Exploiting the Biology of the Child." Moss even plays up the (implausibly) extreme effects of sugar on minorities, saying in the first few pages that food researchers found that "African Americans chose the sweetest and saltiest solutions" in tests of flavor preference. Similarly, *Fed Up* cites the statistic that "one in five Black children ages 2 to 19 is obese, compared with approximately one in seven White children." The parallels are unmistakable. Sugar's origin is morally evil, so it makes sense that it causes physical harm. And if that's not bad enough—just think about how much it harms helpless minorities.

These narratives are powerful, but they distract from a more complicated reality. Difficult though it may be, good science requires us to distinguish between moral evil and physical evil. When we fail to make that distinction, the result is oversimplified myths and cherry-picked facts. Neither *Fed Up* nor *Salt Sugar Fat* mentions that white children consume a higher proportion of their calories in the form of added sugar than black children. Neither mentions that family income is irrelevant to sugar consumption. Those facts, while essential to understanding the complicated relationship between sugar consumption and population demographics, distract from an appealing tale in which sugar does disproportionate harm to poor minorities.

Once people believe in that tale, it becomes very difficult to defend sugar against accusations that it is physically harmful. In the time of Hart and Hanway, skeptics about sugar's harmfulness would have looked like they were defending slavery. Nowadays, the same skeptics—myself included—look like defenders of Big Food and the exploitation of children and minorities. That's good news for anti-sugar alarmists, but not for people who want to know the truth about what we eat.

Nature Really Doesn't Know Best

It took another century before sugar became an issue in America, where marmalades, jellies, sugar candies, and other "confections" were costly imports until at least the 1800s. Shopkeepers like Nicholas Bayard—who opened his New York "Refining House" in 1730—sold their wares only to elites who could afford such extravagant delicacies. Americans were less concerned than the British with the evils of slavery, so there was little reason for them to see refined sugar as harmful—after all, how could something destined for "refined" palates be bad?

That all changed when cheaper sugar put candies within reach of the lower and middle classes. A new kind of shop, the candy store, appeared alongside fine confectionaries. With windows full of brightly colored treats, these candy stores served a new product, penny candy, to a very different clientele. As Wendy Woloson writes in her history of sugar: "Penny candy, more accessible to larger groups of younger people, represented freedom and pleasure to children . . . [it] took refined sugar out of the mouths of the elite and counted among the ways in which sugar, sweetness, and candies became associated with the weak rather than the powerful."

Suddenly moral reformers sprang into action, decrying this new vice with whatever scientific rhetoric they could muster. An early American condemnation of penny candy, written in 1834, provides an amazingly detailed blueprint for anti-sugar advocacy that remains in use today, right down to the use of the word "poison":

> We always regard it as an ill omen when we find the young very fond
> of confectionary. A fondness for fruits is quite a different thing. These

are generally of a cooling nature, and come at a season of the year
when cooling aliments are especially demanded. . . . Taken between
meals, [confectionary] interfere with digestion; taken with our food,
though they may accelerate that process for a time, they weaken the
stomach in the end, and some of them are actually poisonous.

Note the distinction between fruit and candy, a difference observed by almost every anti-sugar advocate throughout history, including the World Health Organization and Dr. Robert Lustig. Who
would listen if someone started bad-mouthing apples? But the distinction, while intuitive, is hard to defend scientifically. The writer
from 1834 appeals to humoral medicine—"a cooling nature"—along
with the seasonality of fruits, which, as dictated by Nature in her
infinite benevolent wisdom, provides them to us when "cooling aliments are especially demanded."

Now humoral medicine is no longer fashionable, and fruits are
available yearlong. So how does a modern man of science like Lustig
explain the difference between fruit and other sugars? By pairing science with an intentional Nature that has our best interests in mind, of
course:

Whereas fruit does contain fructose, it also has inherent fiber. And
that's not by accident. The reason the fructose in fruit doesn't cause
significant health problems is that it's balanced by the endogenous
fiber that makes up the solid part of the fruit. If you consume both
together, as Nature intended, it reduces the rate of flux to the liver;
the liver can keep up, which mitigates most of the negative effects of
the sugar.

One wonders why you couldn't just eat high-fiber bran muffins with
added sugar, if it's fiber that mitigates negative effects of sugar. And
if sugar is so addictive, then why aren't fruits addictive? As Yale

nutritionist Dr. David Katz points out, there's just no logic behind the idea that *"fructose is toxic, except the one place where you will actually encounter it in pure form, namely fruit."*

Lustig's scientific vocabulary can be very convincing, so try to keep in mind what Philip

There's just no logic behind the idea that "fructose is toxic, except the one place where you will actually encounter it in pure form, namely fruit."

Zeitler told me: *Most of what we know about the relationship between sugar, liver metabolism, obesity, and type 2 diabetes remains theoretical.* The only certain metabolic difference between fruit and candy, he assured me, is that it's a lot easier to eat tons of candy than it is to eat tons of apples. Nature's intentions, whether regarding fiber or the seasonality of fruit, are a mark of superstitious hyperbole, not science.

The appeal to Nature with a capital *N* continually wreaks havoc on our ability to objectively evaluate evidence. Take honey and high-fructose corn syrup, two common liquid sweeteners. Seduced by the magic of "natural" origins, countless health articles and blog posts find reasons to distinguish honey from its evil, "artificial" competitor. In *The Healing Powers of Honey*, we read that "honey contains dozens of different substances, which makes it more like fruit than sugar." The author, Cal Orey, tells her readers that she no longer eats yogurt with high-fructose corn syrup, opting instead for plain yogurt with honey on top. And in an article touting the benefits of honey, Paleolithic diet guru Mark Sisson links to a video of a tribesman from the Congo climbing a tree to harvest honey, as if to reinforce the virtue of the substance by highlighting the natural, primal, premodern mode of its cultivation.

"Should you eat it?" asks Sisson, and then proceeds to mask his superstition with scientific rhetoric. "That depends. Are you active and in need of liver glycogen repletion like the guy who climbed the Congolese tree? Then raw honey might be a nice choice for a treat."

Scientists would be surprised to hear about the "clear superiority" of honey, since there is a near unanimous consensus that the biological effects of high-fructose corn syrup are essentially the same as those of honey. But because of its natural origin, honey has enjoyed irrational, superstitious praise from the moment it entered into competition with granular sucrose derived from cane juice. In 1852, physician James Redfield argued in his book *Comparative Physiognomy* that each stage of sugar processing was a "stage in the down-hill course of deception and mockery, of cowardice, cruelty, and degradation." According to Redfield, animals that live on honey are courageous and careful, "as, for example, the bee, the humming-bird, and the bear," while those that prefer sugar are deficient in virtue, "as, for example, the housefly, the ant that lives in the sugar-bowl, and not unfrequently the wasp." Eat natural honey and become like the courageous bear! Eat processed, degraded, modern sugar, and sink to the level of lowly ants and icky wasps.

The public shared Redfield's bias, which meant nineteenth-century sugar companies worked hard to play down the difference between honey and other sweeteners. Henry Tate, the British sugar merchant, went so far as putting a lion carcass swarming with insects on the label of his "Golden Syrup"—still sold today by sugar giant Tate & Lyle, macabre label and all. The carcass refers to a passage from the Bible, Judges 14, where Samson kills a lion and bees make their home in its body. The message of the label is clear, and it echoes the scientific consensus of sugar experts: golden syrup is just like honey.

In a parallel move, the Corn Refiners Association has fought irrational bias against high-fructose corn syrup by lobbying the FDA to rename the sweetener "corn sugar" so people would stop demonizing their product. The image of corn syrup had been smeared through association with soda companies, which made people more likely to believe controversial claims about its health effects. Remarkably, public health advocates agreed.

"I'm not eager to help the corn refiners sell more of their stuff," said Dr. Marion Nestle of New York University, author of *Food Politics: How the Food Industry Influences Nutrition and Health* and generally a staunch opponent of anything the food industry wants. (Remember, she liked Denmark's fat tax.) "But you have to feel sorry for them. Even I have to admit it's not an unreasonable [change]."

Reason and rationality did not rule the day in 1852, and they do not today. In 2012, the FDA—so often accused of being in the pocket of Big Food—ruled that corn syrup cannot be renamed, and many health-conscious consumers will continue to believe, mistakenly, in the mythic goodness of natural honey and the evil of unnatural, processed sugars. In a 2014 blog post about Fig Newtons, the wildly popular Vani Hari, aka "The Food Babe," refers to high-fructose corn syrup as a "toxic processed chemical" and claims it is a "major cause of heart disease, cancer, dementia, and liver failure." Her citation for the claim? An article by none other than Dr. Mark Hyman, titled "Five Reasons High Fructose Corn Syrup Will Kill You"—which runs right next to an advertisement for his books, *The 10-Day Detox* and *The Blood Sugar Solution*.

In a sense, the Food Babe has proved her point—processed sugar really can cause dementia. Thankfully, the antidote is simple: just don't listen to the fearmongers.

Sugar: The New Gateway Drug

Even the rhetoric of addiction can be traced to nineteenth-century America. In *Comparative Physiognomy*, Redfield invoked another popular anti-sugar trope, comparing an appetite for it to alcoholism (instead of cocaine addiction):

The use of sugar is the stepping-stone to intemperance. The appetite grows upon a man by indulgence [. . .] and when the appetite comes upon him, like that of the drunkard for his cups, he wanders and almost rushes in search of it, and goes from one candy-shop to another as the toper goes from one coffeehouse to another to satisfy himself with drams.

Temperance advocates had been against sugar for at least a decade before Redfield's book was published. Their suspicion had its basis in magical thinking: rum was produced from sugar, so sugar shared rum's dangerous properties. It was widely believed that sugar was a gateway drug and a taste for it foreshadowed deadlier habits. This inevitable progression happens to Henry Haycroft, the fictional protagonist of an 1843 temperance tale, who eats "the sugar out of the bottom of his father's toddy-glass," before graduating to real drinks of sweet peppermint cordial shared with friends. "The liquor tasted so sweet," warns the author of the story, "that they all took a large quantity." As one Dr. A. C. Abbott put it in 1907: "The appetite for alcohol and the appetite for candy are fundamentally the same, the choice of the one or the other indulgence being determined by the temperamental qualities of the individual." One addiction easily led to another.

Even then, anti-sugar advocates knew the power of addiction language to motivate outrage. The early temperance movement developed the concept of physical addiction in the process of making alcoholism a medical condition—moving it from "sin" to "sickness." At the end of the eighteenth century, the renowned physician, temperance advocate, and Founding Father Benjamin Rush defined the connection between drinker and distilled drinks as "addiction," a "disease of the will" that developed slowly over time.

The idea of addiction turned demonic possession into a physical condition. Alcoholic spirits stole your willpower, but not via the power of actual spirits. Demons were replaced with terms such as "craving" and "insatiable desire," through which "Demon Rum," as it was called, worked evil on the soul.

By calling addiction a *disease* of the *soul*, temperance advocates combined religious and philosophical fears with physical fears. No one wants a corrupted soul; no one wants to be sick. Alcoholism as addiction made for an enemy as frightening as Satan and as real as cholera, tuberculosis, and yellow fever.

Anti-sugar advocates appropriated this language to create a new disease with no empirical basis: "addiction" to sweets. Along with the new disease came a new set of villains: sweets manufacturers, candy shop proprietors, and, perhaps worst of all, the dreaded operators of ice cream soda fountains. It didn't matter that 2-liter soda bottles hadn't yet been invented—these dens of sin received the same censure that Big Gulps do now. Initially soda fountains were perceived as providing a clean, dainty, ladylike alternative to men's taverns. But before long, reformers swooped in and decried these pleasures as the woman's version of penny candies, corrupting of morals and health, and, of course, as addictive as the alcohol they replaced.

Sex and Candy

It's worth reminding ourselves that all this sucrophobia existed before the epidemic of obesity and type 2 diabetes that animates modern anti-sugar advocates. (Strangely, despite the lack of scientific evidence, people still think diabetes is *caused* by sugar, a belief so prevalent it appears as Myth No. 3 in the American Diabetes Association's myths section.) Instead of obesity, diabetes, and ADHD, nineteenth-century reformers had another set of problems they tried to pin on sugar. While indigestion and general ill health numbered among the negative consequences of consuming candy, ice cream, and soda, most frightening to Puritan anti-sugar advocates was sugar's potential to inflame sexual desire, particularly in the weakest members of society: women, children, and the poor.

Hilariously, ice cream parlors inspired sensational tales of sweet treats leading to licentious behavior. Feed a woman ice cream, went the rumors, and she'll sleep around. Fine chocolates, too, became associated with women's inability to resist temptation, just like the sexually promiscuous, dark-skinned savages who featured, often naked, in early chocolate advertisements.

Luxurious indulgences—that is, sweets—are the "great enemy of [women's] souls," wrote Margaret Coxe in her 1839 book *The Young Lady's Companion*, and it wasn't difficult to guess what she meant. Culinary pleasures and sexual pleasures satisfied the same animal appetites, so it made sense that one would lead to the other. Both John Harvey Kellogg (coinventor of corn flakes) and Graham believed that sugary treats, along with other powerfully flavored foods, caused women and children to masturbate.

"Candies, spices, cinnamon, cloves, peppermint, and all strong essences," claimed Kellogg, "powerfully excite the genital organs and lead to the [solitary vice]." Another reformer, prominent vegetarian physician William Alcott, counseled parents to tell their children about the "penalties which God, in his providence, has annexed to frequent violations of his laws," laws that included a prohibition on the "solitary vice" and "using too much sugar." One can only imagine what these men would have done with brain images that show the same "hedonic pathways" lit up by drugs—and orgasm—are also lit up by sugar. *Scientific proof that eating candy is just like having sex!*

The Failures of Big Sugar

Part of what made reformers' negative depictions of sugar so compelling was that nineteenth-century candymakers did little to convince the public of the contrary. Eager to attract young customers of all income brackets, candymakers used cheap dyes they knew to be poisonous. Woloson reports that as early as the 1830s, the medical journal *The Lancet* carried articles warning about popular British candies, exported to America, that were adulterated with "red oxide of lead, chromate of lead, and red sulphuret of mercury." Candymaking manuals cautioned, unsuccessfully, against using glazed paper infused with poisonous substances, which children would suck on, resulting in "sore mouths or inflamed gums." Meanwhile, racy advertisements featured women feasting on chocolate in paroxysms of delight, or children made crazy by candy cravings. Prefiguring the "cuckoo for Cocoa Puffs" ad campaign, one popular turn-of-the-century confection named Kandi Kubes was advertised with the following rhyme: "Handy-Spandy, Jack-A-Dandy, wants a piece of PEANUT CANDY. He wants it now, he wants it bad, and KANDI KUBES just make him glad."

By the mid-nineteenth century, children could be seen sucking away on candy cigarettes and cigars, sold at combination tobacco-candy stores, where storekeepers not infrequently allowed their youthful customers to purchase real cigarettes. "Kiddie slot machines" enticed youngsters with jackpots of bubble gum. Far from working against the association of sugar and sinfulness, candy marketers recognized the appeal of vice and shamelessly exploited it.

As with modern food companies, the makers of sugary treats in nineteenth-century America didn't do themselves any favors, blatantly disregarding the welfare of their young customers. And like modern anti-sugar advocates, well-intentioned reformers were responding to a host of real and reasonable concerns— among them cavities and rapacious marketing. But good intentions do not redeem bad science. History tells us that if we let missionary zeal bias our perspective on the evidence,

Good intentions do not redeem bad science.

blaming sugar for society's current ills may one day look like blaming sugar for weak nerves and masturbation.

Pure, White, and Biased

Most people are well aware of the bias that can arise from financial conflicts of interest. Scientific journals attempt to counter this bias by having authors disclose those conflicts, which is a good thing.

There is significantly less awareness, however, of what biostatistician David B. Allison calls "white-hat bias": *bias leading to distortion of information in the service of righteous ends*. White-hat bias motivated the anti-sugar advocates of the nineteenth century, and it continues to motivate media, health authorities, and the scientific community.

In a 2009 paper for the *International Journal of Obesity*, Allison and a coauthor demonstrated how white-hat bias affects research on sugar-sweetened beverages. To do so, they began by choosing two studies designed to assess the effect of reducing sugar-sweetened beverage consumption on obesity. Then they looked at how the studies were cited. In the majority of cases, researchers exaggerated the strength of the evidence from the original studies, making it look like reducing soda really helped with obesity, when in fact the evidence wasn't so clear. This is known as "citation bias," which obesity researchers now acknowledge as a problem in their field.

For evidence of white-hat bias in the media, one need only turn to the statistics we saw earlier, cited in the "facts" section of *Fed Up*'s website. Let's start with "One soda a day increases a child's chance of obesity by 60 percent." Scary, right?

Not really. This so-called fact is based on a single 2001 study. The study, published in *The Lancet*, a highly regarded journal, examined self-reported beverage consumption by a group of 548 Boston eleven-year-olds. The children filled out two questionnaires about their sweetened beverage consumption over a thirty-day period, the first in 1995 and the second in 1997. They also filled out questionnaires about physical activity, television watching, and video game playing, so investigators could control for these factors.

And right here, before any discussion of the results, we see evidence of glaring white-hat bias. There was no survey about how much book reading or studying the children did—both sedentary activities. Why? Because "virtuous" sedentary activities are rarely considered as possible contributors to obesity. Does increased homework lead to obesity? Does reading lead to obesity? No one knows, and you'll be hard-pressed to find *any* studies of how book reading or studiousness relates to obesity. The thinking is magical, pure and simple. Just as evil origins create unhealthful products, good activities can't possibly lead to bad consequences. The result is unreliable data, skewed by white-hat bias.

Back to the study. The results of the questionnaires were correlated to BMI. For thirty-seven children, increased servings of sugar-sweetened beverages was predictive of a shift from "not-obese" to "obese," at a rate of 60 percent per serving. (In other words, the odds that someone would go from "not-obese" to "obese" went up by 60 percent per each serving of soda they consumed.) But interpreting this result is not so straightforward. Can we trust the self-reporting of eleven-year-olds? Why did the study consider obesity a categorical variable (yes/no) instead of reporting BMI as a continuous variable? And what about the fact that overall obesity levels for the cohort remained constant, which means thirty-seven children went from obese to not-obese? The reader of the study is left to puzzle over these mysteries.

In science, real science, one thirteen-year-old epidemiological study does not make a fact. The designers of most studies recognize this. The authors of the 2001 *Lancet* paper write in their discussion that the observational nature of the study means it "cannot prove causality." Their findings, far from establishing a fact, can only "suggest that sugar-sweetened drink consumption could be an important contributory factor [to obesity]."

Responsible journalists should follow their lead. But they don't. As Allison points out in his paper, media is often guilty of white-hat bias. Perhaps the most revealing example comes in the *Fed Up* documentary's treatment of Allison himself. First viewers see an ominous image of Allison and learn that he has received substantial industry funding—$2.5 million. (His extensive publication record goes unmentioned, as does his 2009 TOPS research achievement award from the Obesity Society.) Then we see Allison being interviewed. When Katie Couric asks him how he would design a study to examine the relationship of sugar-sweetened beverages to obesity, Allison pauses to collect his thoughts. We never get to hear them, though, because the camera cuts away.

Corruption, pure and simple, the film is telling us. It's trying to show that on one side of this war, led by Couric and Lustig, there is an unbiased army of scientists and reporters courageously fighting against sugar. On the other side are industry stooges like Allison, cooking up terms like "white-hat bias" to defend their corrupt benefactors.

Thankfully there are doctors like David Katz—cited as a consultant for *Fed Up*—who fight against such a simplistic view. After *Fed Up* came out, Katz wrote an entire column defending Allison's research and his credentials.

"Don't private funders want studies to produce a particular outcome?" asks Katz. "Doesn't that introduce bias?" Yes, and yes, he answers. But he adds an important caveat: "What is easy to overlook is that the same is true of all funders, and all researchers."

I asked Katz how he felt about the documentary and its anti-sugar message.

"Their intentions are good, but they are caught up in 'here we are to save the day,'" he says. "And they make the classic New Age mistake with nutrition. There's a colossal problem with focusing on one macronutrient, and with the 'everything you've heard up to now is wrong' message. It perpetuates a vast confusion."

The vast confusion perpetuated by hyperbolic anti-sugar advocacy undermines the credibility of true science, which is humble, cautious, and suspicious of zealotry. Science rejects black-and-white myths starring righteous researchers fighting against toxic substances and evil industries. Science embraces complexity in all its uncertainty and does not lightly pronounce on facts.

To remain unconvinced that one's own pet theory is true takes profound personal strength, particularly when you see how that theory could be deployed to do something good. Sugar may not be evil, but that doesn't mean you should be eating exclusively at McDonald's, supplementing your meals with soda and candy bars—a sobering daily reality for many children. Faced with the enormous marketing power of food companies, medical professionals can be tempted to fight back with whatever they've got.

"If people think foods are addictive, this is something that will get parents upset," Ziauddeen explains during our conversation about sugar's addictive potential. "Researchers I know are open about the idea of food addiction as a way to attack the industry. But I don't think you want to go toe-to-toe with industry based on unfounded science."

Eat Sugar, Stay Sane

And this brings us back to Alice Waters and Edible Schoolyard. If people are really serious about changing food culture, they have to offer a viable alternative. Demonizers of foods don't do that. Instead, they create a hellish world with which we are all too familiar: every food is a potential demon—first fat, then sugar. What next? Talking about food this way is harmful. It creates neurotic eaters who see foods as pure or impure, natural or processed, good or evil. Apple crisps are addictive, poison-filled death traps. Kitchens are stocked with enemies that could do us harm. Restaurants become dangerous battlefields—Lustig writes about how to "survive" going out to eat. Whom can we trust? What can we eat? It's hard to know when every news cycle brings up another scary study and another potential demon.

> **Every food is a potential demon. . . . Talking about food this way is harmful. It creates neurotic eaters who see foods as pure or impure, natural or processed, good or evil.**

Obviously some people enjoy being at war. They enjoy feeling like the good guys in a battle against evil. The world is clearer that way, easier to navigate, and every choice is infused with meaning, purpose, and virtue. Puritans saw sin everywhere—in music, dancing, colorful clothes, and pleasurable food. In a puritanical food world, we see health dangers everywhere. Every culinary choice is filled with meaning, purpose, and virtue, and helps assert control over one's moral and physical destiny. (Remember Vani Hari? She calls her followers "the Food Babe Army.") Sadly, just as there was no evidence of Puritans going to heaven more regularly than anybody else, there is no evidence that living in a food hellscape of demonized macronutrients and toxic chemicals does anything more than make you feel holier-than-thou.

So why not follow a different route? Let's forgo nutrition alarmism and focus on warm, cozy kitchens filled with wonderful smells, kitchens that all good chefs, like the chef teachers at Edible Schoolyard, know should be stocked with pure, white, not-deadly-at-all sugar. Paradoxically, Waters's approach to food feels much healthier than that of *Fed Up*, precisely because it emphasizes joy, not health. The recipes and lesson plans on the Edible Schoolyard website do not include nutrition facts. They focus on how to cook ingredients properly. The ESY "Greens over Grains" sixth-grade lesson plan isn't, as you might think, about the nutritional superiority of greens over grains; it concerns how to sauté greens and serve them over skillfully prepared grains. Sugar features when it should, in desserts like apple crisp.

"We want to slow them down," says chef teacher Esther Cook. "Our students are so stimulated with 'stuff' all day long that they don't always stop and get the feeling of doing ordinary things for pleasure."

This is the same approach taken by America's Test Kitchen, the force behind *Cook's Illustrated* magazine. Jack Bishop, the executive director of America's Test Kitchen, explains to me his team's decision to omit nutritional information from their recipes.

"The numbers are used to demonize individual recipes," he says. "That's not something we want."

It's not just numbers—the very *idea* of sugar as a toxin can demonize recipes, just as it can be used to sell books and documentaries. Thankfully, that idea has no merit. Until the science catches up with the hyperbole, we should join Bishop and Waters and eat our apple crisp (à la mode, even!) guiltlessly, without fear of addiction or impurity. And since there's no evidence that obsessing about sugar leads to better health, slaying this new dietary demon seems like the best way to stop it from making us crazy.

CHAPTER FIVE

The Sin of Salt

How Hard Is It to Limit Your Salt?

Registered dietitian Sharon Salomon always told clients to reduce their sodium to the level recommended by the government. As a trained chef, she assumed her own diet was already in compliance. She cooked all her own meals from scratch. She never ate fast food or packaged snacks. She'd read the studies, like those described in Michael Moss's *Salt Sugar Fat*, which blamed Americans' sky-high sodium consumption on Big Food's salty processed poisons. Surely the FDA's salt guidelines were reasonable, thought Salomon, and only a matter of concern for fast-food junkies, not healthy eaters like herself.

Then she was diagnosed with Ménière's disease. Linked to fluid buildup in the inner ear, symptoms of the disease include hearing loss, dizziness, and nausea. Although there is no cure, standard treatment involves reducing salt intake as much as possible. So Salomon started doing the math—and what she found surprised her. It turned out that the limits on salt proposed by public health advocates and the government were impossibly low—almost at the level recommended for someone with Ménière's. How could that be?

The American Heart Association recommends a daily sodium intake of 1,500 milligrams for everybody, young and old, sick and healthy. (Exceptions are made for super-sweaty people like competitive athletes, foundry workers, and firefighters.) The Centers for Disease Control and the FDA allow more, 2,300 milligrams. But only for 30 percent of the population: African Americans, those with high blood pressure and diabetes, and people over the age of fifty-one should still stick to 1,500 milligrams.

Why the limits? The AHA says that excess salt intake will result in between 500,000 and 1.2 million preventable deaths from cardiovascular disease in America alone. Reducing salt consumption, they claim, will reduce blood pressure, which is linked to poor heart health. If Americans just listened to the AHA's advice, we'd save $26.2 billion in health-care costs. Supposing all of that is true—which it isn't—how hard would it be to comply with their guidelines?

Fifteen hundred milligrams is a big number. It may seem like a generous amount of sodium, but the average American consumes 3,500 milligrams, well over twice that number. Still, average Americans are processed-food addicts, mindless gluttons who might as well be microwaving Cheez Whiz and drinking it from the jar. It's easy to assume that if you just cut out processed snacks and forgo the Bloomin' Onion at Outback, reducing sodium intake is a snap.

Or is it? One teaspoon of table salt contains 2,300 mg of sodium. Just three-quarters of a teaspoon takes you over the AHA's guidelines by 250 milligrams. *Three-quarters of a teaspoon.* Go ahead, measure that out into the palm of your hand. It's shockingly little.

"It is painful," Salomon tells me. "Fifteen hundred milligrams means absolutely, positively never eating out in any restaurant. Unless you can go in and say, 'Please don't salt my water, please don't salt my hamburger, please don't salt my french fries, please don't salt my salad dressing.'"

These guidelines aren't about *added* sodium. They refer to your *total* daily intake. If anything, Salomon is understating the rigidity of the guidelines, which are nearly impossible to follow, even on the most austere of diets. Consider an eating plan advocated by American physician and diet guru John McDougall. Dr. McDougall starts with unprocessed foods direct from nature: starches (like rice and potatoes), vegetables, and fruits. That's around 500 mg of sodium, unless you've splurged and chosen bok choy, carrots, celery, or beets, which push the number higher. Sprinkling a half-teaspoon of salt on these tasty treats adds 1,100 mg of sodium, taking your total daily intake of sodium to 1,600 mg. The plan is extreme: low fat, low sodium, and vegan—and yet it exceeds the AHA maximum.

I'll say it again: a basic diet of starches, vegetables, and fruits, plus *a half-teaspoon of salt*, takes you 100 mg *above* the American Heart Association's recommended daily sodium intake. Add another half-teaspoon of salt and you're over the CDC's generous 2,300 mg allowance.

A basic diet of starches, vegetables, and fruits, plus *a half-teaspoon of salt*, takes you 100 mg *above* the American Heart Association's recommended daily sodium intake.

"Most people haven't even looked at a teaspoon of salt," Salomon says to me. When you put it in your palm and look at it, it's amazing. I can't ever eat Chinese food, which is my favorite."

If 1,500 milligrams now sounds impractically low, you'll find it strange that in 1977, the United States Senate Select Committee on Nutrition and Human Needs told Americans to consume no more than 3 grams of salt per day—which works out to *1,240 milligrams of sodium*!

Following the Committee's guidelines would have required people to abandon any semblance of culinary culture and adopt a radical diet of unsalted fruits, vegetables, starches, and uncured meats.

Such a recommendation could only be justified by overwhelming scientific consensus on the extraordinary health risks of sodium, combined with somber consideration of whether compliance was feasible.

Yet the 1977 guidelines did not reflect overwhelming scientific consensus, and our current 1,500–2,300 milligram limit doesn't either. It's hard to believe that policy makers even tried following their own recommendations. (They certainly don't mention anything about how excruciatingly difficult it is.) Nor, it seems, do they think about the consequences for millions of terrified Americans desperately trying to follow the rules and failing.

The anti-sodium movement owes its success to crusaders and myths, not science. Crusaders, convinced they hold the key to salvation, tend to be impatient, dogmatic, and disinclined to reflect on the negative consequences of what they preach. And myths are compelling in spite of evidence, not because of it. Together, myth and crusading have given us a gospel of impossibly difficult, scientifically groundless guidelines about how much salt to eat.

But fear not. After a good dose of history and skepticism, you'll be guiltlessly sprinkling your food with salt—which, as any good chef knows, will taste a whole lot better than low-salt abominations flavored with dried herbs and lemon juice.

Salt, the Ancient Enemy

In a 2013 commentary for the journal *Epidemiology*, Jiang He and Tanika Kelly of Tulane University assert that the connection between salt and poor health goes back for millennia. They claim that ancient Chinese medical literature connected salt to high blood pressure nearly 5,000 years ago. Their article opens with an impressive quote from the

Huangdi Neijing, aka *The Yellow Emperor's Classic of Internal Medicine*: "Hence if too much salt is used for food, the pulse hardens. . . . "

This line, widely repeated in the literature on salt and blood pressure, has a great deal of persuasive power. Even the ancient Yellow Emperor knew this stuff would kill you! Compelling evidence, right? *Wrong.* Wrong in so many ways.

First: the *Huangdi Neijing* says no such thing. The origin of the quote is actually a 1956 anthology called *Classics in Arterial Hypertension*, compiled by Arthur Ruskin, MD, of the University of Texas. One wonders where Ruskin got the quote, since it's nowhere to be found in the Chinese text. When I checked the original, the only passage that could be construed as referring to high blood pressure—excess *yang qi*—recommended treatment with *increased* salt.

But that's beside the point. The real problem is the inclusion of the quote in a scholarly article. Even if the quote were accurate, it exemplifies a dangerous and deceptive rhetorical device known as the argument from antiquity. Arguments from antiquity carry weight, rightfully, in the realm of theology, where claims can be true simply in virtue of being spoken by ancient prophets or written in revealed texts. Yet in the science of nutrition, the wisdom of Eastern ancients deserves no special attention, unless we are willing to reconsider the medical value of bloodletting, faith healing, and, my personal favorite, "bathing in dog feces to exorcise a demon." The argument from antiquity is just a version of the myth of paradise past. Instead of a long-lost era when people *lived* well, the argument from antiquity appeals to a long-lost era when people *thought* well, romanticizing the wisdom of ancients alongside their lifestyle. Quoting the Yellow Emperor undermines our ability to evaluate evidence objectively.

Learn to ignore these arguments: they are the stock-in-trade of snake oil salesmen. When you don't have real evidence, it's easy to find a version of your pet theory in some old book. Chinese sages with long beards, wise old women prescribing natural folk remedies—these are characters from fairy tales, not trustworthy sources of medical information.

Of course, ancients certainly hit upon some legitimate medical knowledge. Willow bark was used in traditional Chinese medicine to treat pain, and it contains salicin, a chemical similar to aspirin (ace-tyl*salicylic* acid). Galen told his obese patients to eat less. But ancients also filled gaps in their knowledge with demonic possession, astrology, humoral medicine, and countless other principles we have rightfully abandoned.

This isn't the only myth that informs our current restrictive attitude toward salt. Early anti-salt advocacy in America drew on yet another version of the myth of paradise past: *the myth of the noble savage.* Where the argument from antiquity mines the past for wisdom, the myth of the noble savage looks to present-day surviving "primitive cultures" for guidance on how to think and live. By avoiding modernization, noble savages present us with a living embodiment of paradise past. And as it happens, the 1977 salt guidelines issued by the United States Senate Select Committee were inspired in large part by one scientist's belief that noble savages kept their hearts healthy with a low-salt diet. Now we are living with the consequences of wrapping those myths in speculative science.

Let's unwrap them and see how we got here.

A Low-Sodium Miracle

It took a miracle to make people suspicious of salt. Despite the supposed antiquity of salt's connection to high blood pressure, salt was actually a beloved culinary fixture until the mid-twentieth century, playing an indispensible role in food preservation and flavoring across all cultures. Salt also had a distinguished history in medicine. Ancient Greeks and Romans prescribed garum, a salty fermented fish sauce, for digestive disorders, sciatica, tuberculosis, and migraines. Mayans mixed salt with oil to treat epilepsy, and with honey to ease childbirth pains. In the Middle Ages, salt was used to treat toothaches, upset stomachs, and "heaviness of mind."

The first study to suggest salt's darker side came in 1904. Two French physicians, Leo Ambard and Eugene Beaujard, found that increased salt intake in eight of their patients was associated with the retention of sodium and higher blood pressure. Then, in 1920, a clinician named Frederick M. Allen tested the efficacy of salt reduction on twenty of his chronically hypertensive patients and published his results in the *Journal of the American Medical Association*. Allen observed that severely restricting salt provided "great" benefits for hypertension. He also noted that many of his patients had a history of high salt consumption, which further strengthened his hypothesis of a connection between salt intake and high blood pressure. Despite this assessment, Allen sounded a cautionary note that history seems to have ignored: "A diet which is reasonably satisfying and at the same time sufficiently poor in salt is not so easy to arrange as it may appear."

These studies amount to very little. Neither was blinded nor controlled. The sample sizes were extremely small. Consequently, in the years following Allen's work, various articles debated the merits of the sodium–blood pressure connection and judged the evidence inconclusive. A massive, best-selling early-twentieth-century compendium of medical knowledge called *The Library of Health* notes that to treat high blood pressure it is "generally recognized that meats of all kinds should be sparingly eaten and alcoholic liquors should not be used." No mention is made of reducing salt intake—though the authors do suggest using salt to treat toothaches. (They also warn of sugar's toxicity and recommend honey as a healthier alternative.)

The real shift in public and scientific opinions about salt began with news of medical miracles at Duke University Medical Center. On June

12, 1944, the Associated Press reported that Walter Kempner of Duke University had healed the blind and raised the (legally) dead:

> A new entirely drugless treatment for high blood pressure, by a diet of rice and fruit juices, was shown to the American Medical Association today. The diet is mostly rice, boiled or steamed, plus ample fruit juices and supplemented by vitamins and iron.
>
> Many Duke patients were very ill. Some were blind and had enlarged hearts. [...]
>
> There were failures and in one group of 127 patients 16 died. But some successes were spectacular. One patient who was sent to the hospital with autopsy reports already signed, recovered.

At the time, no one had heard of Kempner. Ten years earlier, seeking to escape Hitler's Germany, the thirty-one-year-old physician secured a research faculty position at Duke. During his first few years in America, Kempner practiced English and researched the effect of oxygen deprivation on red blood cells. In the '30s, baby alligators were the best source of cells for that research, and Kempner's assistants occasionally carried them around in their lab coat pockets. The alligators were probably more fun than Kempner, whom one patient would later describe as "a stern dictatorial man, always dressed the same way, in a blue blazer and white ducks—like someone's Nazi grandfather."

Kempner's research on oxygen deprivation led him to develop a theory of kidney failure. Like other cells he studied, kidney cells depended on oxygen for their function, so their dysfunction might be due to reduced blood supply to the kidneys. According to this logic, one possible way to heal kidneys would be by drastically reducing their workload while increasing overall blood flow. This, Kempner suggested, could be accomplished with a diet low in fats and protein— which are difficult for the kidneys to process—and almost no sodium, which some speculated might impede blood flow by increasing fluid retention.

In 1939, Kempner began recruiting patients with cases of chronic kidney disease, and began feeding them his newly formulated "Rice Diet": one small bowl of white rice with a serving of fresh fruit for breakfast, and larger versions of the same for lunch and dinner. Five years later, he presented his results to the American Medical Association in Chicago, accompanied by a battery of x-rays and photographs. Sixty-six swollen hearts reduced. One hundred seven cases of hypertension reversed. Twenty-one cases of retinopathy healed. Of his initial 192-person cohort, twenty-five died and sixty saw no improvement, which sounds bad until you compare his overall results with the typical six-month life expectancy of patients with untreated malignant hypertension.

The AMA did not share the media's initial enthusiasm. Skeptics accused Kempner of falsifying dates, and as a result *JAMA* refused to publish his study. Nevertheless, Kempner's patients vouched for the effectiveness of the Rice Diet, and other physicians tried it out with similar success. In 1946, Kempner presented his results again, this time to the New York Academy of Medicine, where his work was much better received. Though the mechanism of the Rice Diet remained unclear, there was soon no doubt that Kempner's approach resulted in miraculous recoveries for patients with chronic kidney disease.

In this sense, the Rice Diet treatment—and the accounts of miraculous recoveries—resembled Sidney Haas's banana diet treatment for celiac patients. When Hass began his treatment, no one, Haas included, knew exactly why celiac patients recovered on the banana diet, though they did recover quite miraculously. Since Haas believed bananas were the real secret of his diet, the public and physicians jumped to the conclusion that bananas must have health benefits far beyond treating celiac.

Exactly the same thing happened with Kempner's Rice Diet, but with one crucial difference. As soon as a physician named Lewis K. Dahl thought he identified the secret of the Rice Diet in 1950—low sodium—he quickly extrapolated the health benefits of that secret to the general population. But unlike bananas, whose claim to fame depended entirely on their role in treating celiac, Dahl's evangelism of low-sodium diets took strength from the myth of the noble savage. Now, its legacy lives on, in spite of countless skeptical scientists who prefer evidence to myth, and who have found the evidence wanting from the very beginning of Dahl's advocacy.

Salt-Free Noble Savages

In 1950, having heard of the Rice Diet's success, Dr. Lewis K. Dahl of the Rockefeller Institute for Medical Research decided to figure out why it worked. Dahl and his team selected six patients for a six-month continuous residency in a metabolic ward, which gave the investigators full control over the subjects' diets. Although patients remained restricted to rice and fruit, they were allowed to vary their caloric consumption and their sodium intake. After examining the fluctuations in blood pressure experienced by the patients, Dahl saw a clear correlation to sodium intake: more sodium meant higher blood pressure.

Dahl pursued the connection between sodium and hypertension with vigor for the next twenty years. In 1954, he analyzed surveys of "truly primitive human races" and discovered something quite extraordinary. Though they came from radically different environments, the Greenland Eskimo, Australian aboriginal, the mountainous Chinese tribes, and Kuna Indians of Panama all had something in common: virtually no cases of hypertension!

The myth that "savage" races were healthier than civilized folk was already well established. It is, after all, the logical corollary of paradise past: if life was better and healthier in the Garden of Eden, before people were civilized, then uncivilized people should also lead better and healthier lives. Starting in the eighteenth century, the myth of the noble savage colored accounts of Native Americans by physicians like Benjamin Rush, the Founding Father and temperance advocate we met in the previous chapter. Just take a look at Rush's description of childbirth among the "savage" Indians of North America: "Nature is their only midwife. Their labours are short, and accompanied with little pain. Each woman [delivers] in a private cabin, without so much as one of her own sex to attend her. After washing herself in cold water, she returns in a few days to her usual employments." The account is laughably implausible, unless you factor in the Bible, where the pains of childbirth are God's punishment for eating from the tree of knowledge. Of course Rush, a devoutly religious man, was willing to believe that uncivilized, savage women just pop kids out without any pain! (Rush was also one of the first to describe the Native American diet as entirely salt-free, "till they were instructed to [use salt] by the Europeans." This is not entirely true—some North American indigenous peoples actually had salt deities, and salt gathering was a religious ritual.)

By Dahl's time there was widespread disagreement about why primitive people were so healthy. One theory appealed to the simplicity of their lives: live off the grid and you'll feel better. Dahl didn't buy it, and pointed out that savages constantly struggled with famine, fought wars on a regular basis, and lived under the oppressive weight of "taboos and social pressures."

Instead, Dahl saw evidence to confirm his own pet hypothesis. "It was of interest," he wrote in the 1954 article, "to find that a factor common to all the primitive groups for which data were available was a low intake of sodium in the diet." Savages may have been stressed out, but a low-salt diet kept their blood pressure low.

Dahl's article and others that built on it were widely cited and highly influential. In 1969, Dahl appeared before George McGovern's

Select Committee on Nutrition and Human Needs, spinning a tale of saltless savages. Careful not to overstate his case, Dahl still felt justified in recommending policy action on the basis of unsettled science:

> We have evidence which suggests that among societies chronically on a high salt diet, hypertension is much more frequent than among societies in which salt intake is low. Such circumstantial evidence does not alone establish a cause-effect relationship, but in conjunction with other data, it has led us to propose that chronic ingestion of excess salt can play a causal role in human hypertension.

Never mind that Dahl's circumstantial evidence was scientifically flimsy. Never mind the difficulties faced by modern epidemiologists in obtaining reliable blood pressure and dietary data for large populations, much less those who were working in the 1950s with "primitive cultures." And never mind the enormous difference between *treating* hypertension with a low-salt diet and *preventing* hypertension with a low-salt diet. Dahl's noble savages bridged the gap between the two, and a new dietary demon was born.

Save the Children

The circle of salt's potential victims grew at an alarming rate. Part of Dahl's research into the evils of salt involved breeding a strain of salt-sensitive rats, in which he induced hypertension by feeding them commercially prepared baby food that contained added sodium. In April 1970, newspapers ran an Associated Press report about Dahl's findings under scary headlines like "Baby Food Salt May Be Harmful, Researcher Says." The report quoted Dahl calling salted baby food "a needless kind of risk."

But Dahl's opinion was just that—an opinion. Others did not share it: a 1970 National Academy of Sciences committee declared there was "no evidence" in favor of limiting infant salt consumption. Strangely, the absence of evidence didn't stop academy members from suggesting that added salt be restricted in baby food. Though a harmless action in itself, the suggestion reinforced the dangerousness of salt in the public eye—just as the National Research Council's suggestion to eliminate MSG from infant formula did for MSG in the very same year.

Seven years later, Senator McGovern convened the "Diet Related to Killer Diseases" nutrition hearings. Largely on the strength of Dahl's research, the hearings resulted in the nation's first recommended daily allowance of salt: just one half-teaspoon per day. Given the perceived danger to children, the recommendation was politically expedient, if not scientifically justified. And again, just like with MSG, companies caved to market pressures despite lack of evidence. In 1977, Baker/Beech-Nut revealed a new line of "natural baby foods" free of added salt, and Heinz followed suit by eliminating added salt from all 108 of its baby food varieties.

Dietary Demon Déjà Vu

The ensuing history of salt's demonization recapitulates practically every nutrition myth imaginable. One way of attacking salt has been to describe our appetite for it as "unnatural," yet another variation on the myth of paradise past. In line with anti-sugar and anti-grain advocates, anti-salt advocates argue that evolution fine-tuned our ancient ancestors to live in a naturally salt-poor environment. Like Dahl's present-day savages, these ideal, primitive humans enjoyed good health and low blood pressure until modernity yanked them out of their natural paradise. When salt became artificially abundant as a product of civilization, everything went to hell. In the words of a 1978 article from the *American Journal of Clinical*

When salt became artificially abundant as a product of civilization, everything went to hell.

Nutrition: "Throughout man's history salt was scarce and man would never have survived without the development of regulatory mechanisms for retaining salt in his body. It has only been within the last few hundred years that salt has been abundant. The human body was not equipped to handle the unnatural amount of sodium in the diet."

Aligned with this myth was the alarming idea that children are born innocent of a taste for salt, only to be corrupted by our evil, modern world. Noble savages and primitive people maintain their innocence—and their health—by avoiding civilization. Children born into our toxic modern times are not so lucky. In *Salt Sugar Fat*, Michael Moss echoes the 1978 study, parlaying the notion of an acquired taste for "supranormal" amounts of salt into a sinister portrait of processed-food companies poisoning youngsters and defiling their natural tendencies. Kids are not born liking salt, Moss stresses. They are *taught* to like salt by greedy corporations, and once they are six months old their depravity knows no bounds. Salt addiction drives them to "lick salt from the surface of foods" and even "eat plain salt."

As we have now come to expect, this story of a dietary fall from grace needs a Satan, and anti-salt advocates found theirs, as usual, in the food industry. Yet again there appeared the familiar and deceptive analogy to tobacco. Lewis Dahl himself compared the relationship between cigarette smoking and cancer to that of salt and hypertension as early as 1970. During the 1980s, British newspapers uncovered industry-funded studies of salt and political manipulation. And in 1996, associate editor of the *British Medical Journal* Fiona Godlee effectively labeled all anti-salt skeptics as industry stooges. "The food industry has everything to gain from keeping the controversy alive," she wrote. "But if [the British government] is serious about reducing premature deaths from cancer and heart disease it will need to ignore the voices of vested interest and listen to the advice of its independent experts."

As recently as September 2014, Marion Nestle of NYU continued the tradition, attacking an editorial published by Dr. Suzanne Oparil in the *New England Journal of Medicine*. Oparil, writing about three new studies, concluded that "the results argue against reduction of dietary sodium." Nestle knew that couldn't be true; the evil food industry was obviously to blame. Rather than addressing Oparil's points, she invoked the mythic battle between Big Food and innocent consumers.

"Although Dr. Oparil reports receiving grants or fees from companies making anti-hypertensive drugs—and, even more remarkable, from the Salt Institute—she states that she has no conflicts of interest," wrote Nestle on her blog. "I think she does."

The Bias Is Back

When it comes to salt, Godlee and Nestle are misled by the same white-hat bias that leads to irrational demonization of sugar. They seek to validate a myth in which anti-salt skeptics are minions of evil industry, and anti-salt advocates are unbiased and good. Yet ever since Dahl first suggested a causal connection between salt consumption and hypertension, the connection has met with stiff, nonpartisan, science-based resistance. Work continued to be done that lent credibility to both sides of the debate. One of the most important studies in this regard was the 1988 Intersalt study, which examined 10,079 people from thirty-two countries. The results were first discussed in the *British Medical Journal*, and experts drew diametrically opposed conclusions from the same data, a common occurrence in the world of nutrition science.

The Intersalt researchers themselves reported a correlation between low salt consumption and low blood pressure. But their report ran alongside a rebuttal by John Swales, founding editor of the *Journal of Hypertension*. Swales called the correlations "weak," contrasted the ambiguity of salt's effects with the unambiguousness of alcohol's, and said he hoped the data would help restrain the "evangelical fervour" of anti-salt advocates.

"We should guard against giving prescriptive advice," Swales warned, "based on weak epidemiological relations. [. . .] Doctors should not engage in an intellectual lobotomy that equates statistical significance with biological, physiological, or quantitative importance."

But people want to know what they should eat, and the desire to be purified, saved from disease and death, leads us to demand—and discover—rules that go beyond what the evidence warrants. These rules are reinforced by myths—of evil corporations, noble savages, and paradise past—and promulgated by evangelists.

The truth is far more complicated. There's no doubt that industry creates biased research. Nevertheless, research universities can also be "self-interested." So can individual scientists, whose desire to uncover new truths may lead to biased interpretations of their own data. Industry lobbies influence science and public policy, and that's a bad thing. But dismissing all science that aligns with industry interests allowed—and continues to allow—opponents of salt to ignore legitimate dissent.

Regardless, legitimate dissent most definitely exists, independent of industry pressure. In 1998, Gary Taubes brought that dissent to light in a blistering exposé for *Science* titled "The (Political) Science of Salt." After extensive interviews and research, Taubes concluded that there was, indeed, a serious lack of scientific consensus on the effects of salt, harmful or otherwise.

Part of the problem, he argued, was the intuitive physiological plausibility of the case against salt: Eat more salt and your body will retain more water to maintain homeostasis. Water retention, in turn, leads to an increase in blood pressure, which provides a simple explanation of the connection. But as Taubes noted, the homeostatic mechanism that regulates blood pressure is actually immensely complex and poorly understood. Nearly twenty years after his article, theories about how salt affects this homeostasis remain highly speculative. In 2012, researchers from Boston University concluded that "salt-induced hypertension is not attributable to intravascular fluid expansion"—a complete departure from the water retention hypothesis. Articles published in the years since entertain a variety of alternative theories, none of which are anywhere near conclusive.

The medical effects of salt have been and still are a matter of debate. In an exhaustive 2012 survey of the salt wars, cowritten by an epidemiologist and two sociologists of health at Columbia University, the authors conclude that scientific uncertainty about salt has been systematically left out of policy decisions, a "mistake that serves neither the ends of science nor good public policy." And in August 2014, the *New York Times* ran an article by Dr. Aaron Carroll, professor of pediatrics at Indiana University, in which he examined new studies about sodium and concluded there was "surprisingly little rationale" for current salt guidelines—the same conclusion arrived at by industry-funded Suzanne Oparil, whom Nestle criticized as biased.

Meanwhile, organizations like the AHA and the CDC have kept their low-sodium recommendations unchanged in the face of contradictory evidence. As of September 2014, for example, the CDC recommends that all adults age fifty-one or older and all African Americans reduce sodium intake to 1,500 mg. They recommend this despite a 2013 study by the Institute of Medicine, *commissioned by the CDC itself*, which found no evidence in favor of treating the elderly or African Americans any differently than the rest of the population. The recommendations remain in

Organizations like the AHA and the CDC have kept their low-sodium recommendations unchanged in the face of contradictory evidence.

place despite the IOM having found no evidence that reducing sodium below 2,300 milligrams is beneficial for anyone. And they remain in place despite a 2014 Canadian study that found the safest levels of sodium consumption are between 3,000 mg and 6,000 mg. Even more worrisome, both the Canadian study and the IOM study concluded that eating too little sodium—the amount recommended by the CDC and the AHA—could in fact *increase* risk of cardiovascular problems! (Americans consume, on average, 3,400 mg, toward the lower end of the safe spectrum, and well below the global average of 3,950 mg.)

So why don't the CDC and the AHA admit uncertainty, even at the potential cost of public health? Perhaps because dictating dietary rules, a sacred role that was once the province of priests, contributes to a savior complex. Saviors must remain unwaveringly certain about their mission. They cannot reverse positions, because doing so undermines their authority in the eyes of their followers. And in the case of dietary rules that require substantial willpower to follow—like drastic reductions in sodium—any uncertainty on the part of dieters can lead to failure. Better to conceal scientific ambiguity than to compromise the willpower of your followers.

Dietary gurus' savior complexes get far less attention than food industry conflicts of interest, but they can be just as dangerous. Even the best scientists and institutions are susceptible. For an extreme case, just look at Walter Kempner, the Duke University miracle worker and founder of the Rice Diet. He, too, had an undeclared conflict of interest.

The God of Fat City

After treating chronic kidney failure with the Rice Diet, Kempner became well known in the medical community. True celebrity status, however, resulted from a side effect of the Rice Diet: extreme weight loss. Within a matter of years, the bulk of visitors to Kempner's clinic were there to slim down. Kempner became known as the Rice Diet

Doctor, his monastic regime endorsed by a raft of cultural icons, among them performer Burl Ives, comedian Buddy Hackett, trumpeter Al Hirt, Mario Puzo, Dom DeLuise, numerous NFL players, and even Supreme Court Justice Stanley Reed. Household names praised Kempner's methods on *The Tonight Show* and in the pages of *Ladies' Home Journal* and *Good Housekeeping*.

By 1960, the wildly popular Rice Diet Center had earned Durham, North Carolina, the nicknames "Fat City" and "Diet Capital of the World." It also earned Duke University millions of dollars, not including the $8 million that Kempner donated to the medical center in early 1997, just months before he died. County officials estimated that the Rice Diet contributed up to $30 million annually to the local economy. So many dieters—"Ricers"—flocked to the city that residents referred to planes as "flab flights" and the pool at Duke Towers Apartments as "Whale Watch."

But in October 1997, Kempner's posthumous status as a beloved weight-loss guru and champion of the connection between sodium and hypertension was suddenly in jeopardy. Newspapers across the nation picked up a shocking story of abuse and brainwashing that had first come to light in 1993, when former patient Rebecca Reynolds sued Kempner for malpractice. Her complaint was not the first. Indeed, it came out that in 1975, allegations by other patients led the vice president for health affairs at Duke Hospital to quickly and quietly ban Kempner from the premises, nevertheless maintaining their financial relationship. The cover-up worked, and Kempner suffered no further repercussions until Reynolds decided to speak up.

And speak up she did. Her affidavit described how she came to the Rice Diet Center in 1970, insecure and overweight, only to be forced by Kempner into the position of a "virtual sex slave/servant." For the first five months, everything had gone well, and the twenty-year-old Reynolds dropped 50 pounds. But then she gained a little weight. When he found out, Kempner allegedly instructed her to remove her pants and underwear and then whipped her with a riding crop. (In his deposition Kempner admitted to whipping a number of women, including Reynolds, but insisted they asked for it.)

"I was crying because I thought I was bad, deserved to be whipped," said Reynolds in her affidavit. "By this point I believed Kempner could do no wrong, and I was grateful for Dr. Kempner's concern and care for me."

Reynolds was not alone in her worship. Kempner never married, instead cultivating a circle of a dozen adoring women composed of former patients, employees, and acquaintances from his native Germany, some of them doctors. There was the young, beautiful brunette Fides Ruestow, psychologist Mercedes Gaffron, and gynecological surgeon Dr. Christa von Roebel, who left her husband behind in Germany to join Kempner in 1949.

The women's houses, subsidized or purchased outright by Kempner, were connected by walkways that allowed them to visit each other with ease. They gathered regularly at Kempner's residence to sit at his feet and listen as he expostulated on philosophy or art. Their adulation of the doctor was disturbingly intense. On holidays Reynolds brought him bowls of whipped cream—forbidden to her, of course. She gave him a gold box with seventy-seven sapphires on his seventy-seventh birthday. For his eightieth, she rented out Duke's football stadium and staged a fireworks show. According to the deposition of Joanne Passaro, a former Ricer, all the members of this inner circle, or "Kreis," would refer to Kempner in letters and notes as "He" or "Him" with a capital *H*. In their wills they named Him as their heir.

Kempner's charismatic power was not limited to his Kreis. It extended to the entire Ricer community. "He was everyone's most beloved, most powerful person," said Passaro. "Nobody would make a movement without him. [. . .] He was truth, capital *T*; Light, capital *L*."

Other accounts confirm her testimony. In her book *Fat Like Us*, folklorist Jean Renfro Anspaugh recalled Kempner's domineering personality. "Dr. Kempner was the program's total and absolute head," she wrote. "His authority was supreme. As he told one potential Ricer, 'If I ask you to eat wallpaper, you will eat wallpaper.'"

The savior complex so evident in Kempner's relationship with his Ricers also affected his relationship with fellow scientists. Having discovered an effective treatment, Kempner had no patience for skeptics and brooked no dissent about the details of his diet. Many people made reasonable complaints: Kempner refused to use control groups, for instance, which made it difficult to isolate his diet's mechanism. Was it weight loss? The absence of sodium? The peculiar combination of fruit juice and white rice? But Kempner didn't care for the scientific method. Citing a deep love for his patients, he argued that there was no need to investigate any further. Doing so would simply mean that some people would be forced to miss out on a clearly effective treatment.

For researchers intent on employing the scientific method, Kempner's attitude was alienating. But at Duke, where the money and accolades were pouring in, colleagues were impressed. Dr. Eugene Stead, the chairman of Duke's Medical Center and founder of the physician assistant profession, praised Kempner for refusing to appeal to the scientific community.

The problem is that a love of patients is not a love of truth. In Kempner's case it constituted an egregious conflict of interest. Such evangelical fervor can cause diet gurus to ignore the potential harmfulness of their advice: harm to patients who can't stick with the diet, and to patients who stick with it by adopting a cultish mentality. Regarding these potential harms, the AHA and the CDC should think hard about what happened to Kempner's Ricers before recommending their own draconian rules.

The Low-Salt Cult

For a good look at what happened to Fat City visitors, there is no better book than *Fat Like Us*, a combination memoir and set of interviews by Jean Renfro Anspaugh, herself a former Ricer. Reading *Fat Like Us*, it is impossible to ignore the deep religiosity that infused every aspect of a Ricer's life. The journey to Durham was a "pilgrimage," a response to "the Call" that involved immense personal sacrifice. Food itself was imbued with talismanic power, "divine" and "mysterious." Kempner told his patients that no sacrifice was too great for the privilege of being on the Rice Diet, occasionally recommending (tongue in cheek?) that they rob a bank if they ran out of funds. Some patients sold their homes to finance their stay. Many Ricers left behind friends, family, and jobs.

They also left behind the foods they loved. In recognition of this tremendous sacrifice, Ricers prefaced their journey with a ritual known as the Last Supper, during which they would gorge on fat, salt, and sugar, all of which would soon be forbidden. Some had parents or spouses prepare a beloved family dish. Others went to a favorite restaurant. One on-and-off dieter named Sylvia Goldman described how she prepared for an attempt at the Rice Diet by making a list of forbidden foods. "I put all ethnic food on the list," she recounted, "as well as all salty food, because salt is strictly forbidden on the Rice Diet and it is what I miss the most." The Rice Diet involved complete separation from one's previous food culture and community.

Like Frederick M. Allen in 1920, Kempner knew it was exceedingly difficult to create a "reasonably satisfying diet" that is at the same time "sufficiently poor in salt." So he didn't try. Ricers were allowed four kinds of food: white rice, fruit, and occasionally juice or table sugar. That's it. No salt. No dairy. No meat. No vegetables. For months and months. (Additional supplements provided needed nutrients.)

Strict Buddhist monks allow themselves greater culinary variety. And in order to maintain their diet, that's essentially what the Ricers became:

religious devotees. The Rice Diet Center ritualized the sinfulness of salt and the absolute authority of Kempner over his patients' lives, without which their willpower would certainly fail them. Every day Ricers stepped on the scale, had their blood pressure checked, and, most important, reviewed their sodium counts. The Center displayed these numbers publicly, circling low sodium counts in red. Receiving your first red circle was known as having your cherry popped. Kempner believed all dieters were liars and cheats, so he insisted on twice-weekly urine analyses to make sure no one was sneaking salty foods. Salt became a potent symbol of failure, its presence in one's body cause for overwhelming guilt.

Although Ricers missed high-fat foods, it was the absence of salt that was most painful and alienating. They referred to eating forbidden foods—which meant anything that wasn't sanctioned by Kempner—interchangeably as "sin" or "picking up salt." The dangers of picking up salt were reinforced by legends of former Ricers who ate off the diet and ended up dying.

Improvements in weight and blood pressure notwithstanding, the result of all this, as one might imagine, was an incredibly unhealthy psychological relationship to food. The level of repression required by the Rice Diet is best illustrated by stories of those who sinned:

> The first time I cheated was at Taco Bell. Mexican food is the worst possible choice for a cheat because it is loaded with salt. I decided to have just one bean burrito. The next thing I knew I was ordering three burrito supremes, nachos, refried beans, a king-size Pepsi, and everything else on the menu. The girl at the window couldn't believe it. I told her I was having a party. Cost me over three hundred dollars. I pulled into the parking lot and spent forty-five minutes just gorging on food. Food was flying all over the car. Even the windows were spattered with food. There was taco sauce, hamburger, and dripping cheese everywhere. I looked like I had been in a bad car wreck.

I ordered two extra-large hand-tossed Meat Lovers pizzas with extra cheese and two pitchers of beer. I had the waitress bring everything up on the table at once. I took such pleasure in just looking at all of the fat, greasy, salty food. I scarfed those pies down without actually tasting them and drained both pitchers. All I tasted was the salt and I knew my salt-deprived body was just soaking it up like a sponge. I didn't care. Nothing could stop me from that binge.

More unsettling than the stories of failure are the success stories, which Anspaugh collects in a section of *Fat Like Us* called "Diet Worship." Long-term Rice Dieting required people to divide the world "into what is acceptable and what is taboo." Anything outside of the Rice House "is part of the fallen world." Even from beyond the grave, Dr. Walter Kempner served as "the hierarchal god of the Rice Diet," whose "teachings and proverbs" formed a way of life and "code for proper behavior, much like the Bible or the Koran." Foods low in sodium and calories were seen as sacred and magical. Ricers came to view triumph as a mark of "sainthood," and "cheaters as sinners."

This transformation could result in complete alienation from one's previous community. One Ricer told Anspaugh, "My family and old friends have nothing much to do with me. Some of them think I am a religious zealot because of my eating and exercise habits. I am very faithful to my regimens. They aren't *my* regimens, but those of Dr. Kempner. Remember when he used to tell us that the only way to keep weight off was to remind ourselves each day that we are different from other people . . . ? It is the absolute truth."

Any amount of doubt in their savior was intolerable, because it could lead Ricers into deadly temptation. "I believe in the infallibility of the Rice Diet," said one diet worshipper named Rhonda Beru. "Everything that Dr. Kempner said is true." Beru and countless other converts extolled the singular virtues of the Rice Diet, which, they testified, had transformed them into new people after all else failed. No more medication.

No more arthritis. No more pain. Sharpened mental abilities. "I wake up in the morning with a sense of power and health. I am this way because I adhere to the Diet and have done so for twenty-five years."

Admittedly the meager 150 milligrams of sodium allowed on the Rice Diet is extreme. Ricers like Beru provide a cautionary example of dietary craziness, but they don't tell us what it takes to keep your sodium at the AHA's recommended level of 1,500 mg per day. Is that anything like Kempner's ascetic lunacy?

A Nation of Ricers

Just after the Intersalt study came out, *Vogue*'s Jeffrey Steingarten wrote an essay in 1990 complaining about the hysterical anti-salt environment in America. Was it even possible for anyone to follow the government's salt recommendations? Dutifully, Steingarten tried out a number of recipes from low-salt cookbooks. Verdict? "The food tastes mainly of herbs, spices, garlic, and onions instead of what you wanted for dinner in the first place."

Steingarten's complaints don't go far enough. He points out that gourmet chefs—untainted, one assumes, by the nefarious processed-food industry—insist on the culinary value of salt. But what he doesn't point out, and what dietitian Sharon Salomon discovered at the beginning of this chapter, is that keeping one's sodium intake to 1,500 mg would require the kind of devotional attitude exhibited by Ricers. It doesn't just mean cutting out processed meats and fast food. It doesn't just mean eating out less often. Keeping to 1,500 mg means a monkish isolation from anything remotely resembling an existing food culture. It means becoming a cult member.

Keeping to 1,500 mg means a monkish isolation from anything remotely resembling an existing food culture. It means becoming a cult member.

In 2011, *Washington Post* food writer Tim Carman decided to try reducing his salt to 1,500 mg, in honor of the new 2010 US Dietary Guidelines. He described his effort as a "masochistic experiment" requiring "endless vigilance." Restaurants didn't have sodium information readily available. Nor did food vendors at his local farmers' market. Even chain restaurants referred him to their websites. His advice: trust no one, especially chefs, whose dishes can nail you with half of your daily salt. During his week of salt deprivation, Carman found solace in an "equilibrium of sins," by which he meant drinking more wine than he ever had before.

The difficulty of sticking to a low-salt diet has empirical support. In 2011, *Cochrane Reviews* published a meta-analysis of dietary interventions about salt. The results of the study were widely misreported as confirming that cutting salt has no effect on mortality and heart health. In fact, what the study analyzed was the efficacy of *dietary interventions* to reduce salt intake across populations. While the report tentatively suggested that significant salt reduction *might* be beneficial, attempts to implement that reduction "generally required considerable efforts" and "would not be expected to have major impacts on the burden of cardiovascular disease." In other words: Without Kempner around to whip you, recommendations to reduce salt will only result in increased guilt. And in light of the most recent studies, unless you are consuming twice the amount of salt that average Americans do, your efforts will most likely result in no health benefits—though the guilt-induced stress may strain your heart.

The AHA, the CDC, and other low-sodium advocates ignore all this. Instead, they adopt a jaunty, cavalier tone about the ease of salt reduction, playing up the notion that a taste for salt is unnatural. (Remember the natural, noble savages? Remember the innocent children?) "Many of us have developed a preference for salty flavours due to years of eating manufactured foods with a high salt content," says

Action Salt of Britain, engineers of a nationwide anti-salt movement. "Taste food as it really should taste," reads one of their posters. (Chefs all over England no doubt cringed when they saw it.) The American Heart Association's website is no better. "Change your salty ways," it advises, calling salt the "silent killer" that "slinks into soups and sandwiches and cozies up to cold cuts and cured meats."

Apparently none of these organizations consulted with chefs or historians of food, who would be happy to extol the virtues of salt, along with its ubiquity in world cuisine. Nor, for that matter, did they consult with scientists about the near impossibility of changing your salty ways. Had Steingarten written his essay today, he might have referenced a study that came out in the March 2013 edition of the journal *Nutrition Research*, titled, straightforwardly, "Food pattern modeling shows that the 2010 Dietary Guidelines for sodium and potassium cannot be met simultaneously." For the study, three French researchers tried to see if it was actually possible to get your minimum daily intake of potassium while keeping to your maximum daily sodium intake. Their conclusion? It was nearly impossible. "Even after reducing the sodium content of all US foods by 10 percent," the authors wrote, "modeling analyses showed that the 2010 Dietary Guidelines for sodium were incompatible with potassium guidelines and with nutritionally adequate diets." Whether or not we really need our minimum daily intake of potassium, creating incompatible rules is a bad idea.

The CDC's and AHA's salt recommendations are the height of policy irresponsibility. They disguise the controversy behind their numbers and set extraordinarily high bars without considering the consequences. The result is a public frightened of what we put into our mouths, incapable of seasoning food properly, paranoid about what we are served when eating out or at a friend's home. Even if the alarmist claims about salt proved true, it would require an entirely new food culture to comply with the health commandments we've been given.

All elimination diets run the risk of turning us into a nation of Ricers, devoted to salvific food, incapable of questioning the authorities that have commanded us to eat that way. We suffer while the food industry prospers, developing religiously themed food products like Hormel's "Sin Free" line of low-calorie, reduced-sodium desserts and "Guiltless Gourmet" unsalted potato chips.

That's a terrible, dystopian world. We don't want to infuse food, as Ricers did, with moral overtones. Salt is part of a pleasurable meal, not a potential agent of damnation. We don't need to steadfastly track our sodium consumption and write it down, as the AHA suggests, on a "Sodium Tracker" sheet, circling good days in red. The destination of that road is ending up like Ricer Jean Renfro Anspaugh, who writes with regret that "to eat with pleasure is something I will never experience again except in stolen moments, and even then it is with the guilt and knowledge that I will pay for each swallow."

As with gluten, there is a small minority of people that need to watch their salt—people like Sharon Salomon who have Ménière's, or those who have a condition known as "salt sensitivity," where small amounts of sodium cause large upward swings in blood pressure. But for the rest of us average Americans, reducing salt makes about as much sense as going gluten-free if you don't have celiac disease. So toss a little salt over your left shoulder, a little more on your food, and rest assured that science—and, more important, your sanity—blesses every bite you take.

CHAPTER SIX

Nutrition Myth Detox

Do You Drink Magical Elixirs?

It's time to revisit the Daoist masters from earlier in the book. Like today's diet gurus, the grain-free monks of ancient China were obsessed with avoiding illness and living forever, and they believed proper eating was the key to both. But back then, like today, no one could agree on what constituted proper eating. Monks recommended grain-free diets, meat-free diets, alcohol-free diets, and even food-free diets, claiming to survive entirely on water and air. And like most of today's diet gurus, they endorsed a variety of dubious dietary supplements: peach sap, coptis root, cassia root, "stony honey," *fuling* fungus, pine resin, the "five metals," the "eight minerals." These were often used as ingredients in health-food recipes, like this one for "Master Halewind's Elixir":

> It is prepared by taking some blood from the chick in a crane's egg and the juice of aconite from the Lesser Chamber and mixing them to

make the elixir. Place in a swan's egg, seal with lacquer, and submerge in mica solution.

Sure, Master Halewind's elixir isn't easy to make, and it probably doesn't taste great. But according to ancient testimonials, drinking "a gill" of it increases your longevity by a hundred years; a quart will increase it by a thousand. In addition to increasing your life span, Daoist elixirs supposedly granted incredible vision, preserved young-looking skin, and expelled "the Three Worms."

This kind of nonsense belongs in a fantasy world. Yet even today, under the influence of myths and superstitions dressed up as science, otherwise reasonable people continue to believe in miracle elixirs just as nonsensical as Master Halewind's.

Take Bulletproof® Coffee, cooked up by self-proclaimed "bio-hacker" Dave Asprey, a beverage many Paleolithic dieters swear by. The recipe:

> Brew 1 cup of coffee using filtered water, with freshly ground Bullet-proof® Coffee Beans. Add in 1–2 tablespoons of Brain Octane® to the hot coffee (It's STRONG—start with 1 tsp. and work up over several days). Add 1–2 tablespoons grass-fed, unsalted butter or ghee. Mix it all in a blender for 20–30 seconds.

Asprey has claimed that normal coffee is loaded with "toxins" that "steal your mental edge and actually make you weak," whereas "clean coffee actually fights cancer and provides antioxidants," bestows "powerful energy and rock steady focus," and "programs" your body to "burn fat for energy all day long," allowing you to "lose 100 pounds without using exercise" and "upgrade your IQ by more than 12 points." (Incidentally, *The Bulletproof Diet* is published by Rodale Books—"I will live to be a hundred!" *cue heart attack*—and enthusiastically endorsed by Dr. Mark Hyman.)

If you buy into food myths, this is the kind of life you can end up living: Scared that your coffee, along with the rest of your food, is filled with toxins. Seeking refuge from the modern world in the reassuring illusion of Paleolithic living. Hopeful that some biohacking savior will tell you how to make genuine cave-brewed java, the kind of java that Java Man would have made for himself—the coffee *we are evolved to drink*! Shelling out money for something called Brain Octane®.

Don't buy into the hype. Keep an eye out for the myth of paradise past. Remember—*you are what you eat* is a superstition, not a fact. Beware of Nature worship. Understand that bias extends beyond industry to individual researchers and diet gurus selling books. Be skeptical of the noble savage. Don't drink the Kool-Aid—or the Bulletproof® Coffee.

Not only will you relax about gluten, fat, sugar, and salt, but you will also be able to defend yourself against new nutritional nonsense—and the next diet or health fad that could cost you money and waste your time.

Superfoods? Superstupids!

Sometimes the nonsense isn't quite as obvious as it is with Bulletproof® Coffee. Maybe Brain Octane® is BS, but what about superfoods like goji berries—aren't they chock-full of cancer-preventing antioxidants?

Short answer: nope. With *every* so-called superfood, it's always the same story: overhyped, under-researched, superstitious nonsense, hidden under scientific rhetoric.

Here's how it happens. According to *Men's Health* magazine, goji berries have one of the "highest ORAC ratings—a method of

With *every* so-called superfood, it's always the same story: overhyped, under-researched, superstitious nonsense, hidden under scientific rhetoric.

gauging antioxidant power—of any fruit, according to Tufts University researchers." They've been used as a "medicinal food in Tibet for over 1,700 years." And "the sugars that make goji berries sweet reduce insulin resistance—a risk factor of diabetes—in rats."

At this point alarm bells should be ringing. Paradise past, this time in Tibet. Claims of extraordinary medicinal power for a single food. If something seems suspicious to you, that's good. For true believers in these little red berries, the history of goji is a real downer.

In *The Fruit Hunters*, journalist Adam Leith Gollner documents how a man named Earl Mindell single-handedly managed to make goji berries magical. Mindell, a veteran of the miracle dietary cure genre (his books, including *Earl Mindell's Soy Miracle* and *Earl Mindell's Vitamin Bible*, have sold millions of copies), published a pamphlet in 2003 called *Goji: The Himalayan Health Secret*. That document introduced the world to the benefits of a superfood now endorsed by Oprah and available at any health food store.

In it, Mindell tells the story of Li Qing Yuen, a Chinese man who used goji berries to live from 1678 to 1930—252 years. The powers of goji berries, writes Mindell, have been confirmed by tests of "infrared molecular bonds" and "spectroscopic fingerprinting." Those powers could have been drawn directly from a Daoist monastic manual, or the cover of *Men's Health*: longevity, virility, fewer headaches, night vision. How long would you like to live, asks Mindell: "Eighty years? Ninety? One hundred-plus years? Perhaps forever?" While writing *The Fruit Hunters*, Gollner tried repeatedly to contact "Dr." Earl Mindell to ask him about these claims. Mindell, whose doctorate comes from the unaccredited University of Beverly Hills, was impossible to locate. The employer listed in his bio, Pacific Western University, denied that Mindell had ever worked for them.

There's a miracle here, all right, but it's not the berry. The miracle is that we keep believing in miracle foods originated by fraudsters like Earl Mindell, and popularized by icons like Oprah and disgrace-ful physicians like Dr. Oz, whose endorsements do more damage to our national mental health than any of the "toxins" he warns against. Superfoods don't have the power to "boost your immune system" or "supercharge your brain." But the myths and superstitions that recur in the histories of gluten, fat, sugar, and salt clearly have the power to make us super-stupid, ready and willing to believe in Himalayan lon-gevity secrets.

In fact, I almost forgot to mention that the Himalayas are the source of another dietary fad. As reported in *Men's Journal*:

> Dave Asprey is a Silicon Valley entrepreneur and leader in the "bio-hacking" movement. . . . Asprey had the idea [for Bulletproof Cof-fee] in Tibet when, exhausted from hiking in the Himalayas, he was treated by some locals to a tea creamed with yak butter. He felt imme-diately revitalized.

Tale Type:
"Toxic Additive Produced by Synthesizing Seaweed"

Now that you know the history of nutrition myths, you'll be surprised how easy it is to identify new ones for what they truly are. The same themes pop up again and again: the same emphasis on good and evil, the same false promises, the same superstitions. Sometimes you'll even see the exact same plot, modified very slightly in its details.

Scholars of folk and fairy tales call this kind of repeated story a "tale type." There are general categories for tale types—like "animal tales" or "religious tales"—within which there are more specific subcategories, such as "the clever fox" and "man outwits the devil."

If folklorists focused on what we eat, they could add a whole new category: food tales. In this category we'd find subcategories like "miracle food from Tibet" and "dietary cures for chronic disease" and "everyday

food is actually poisonous." I, for one, think the public would benefit from this addition to folklore studies. Instead of feeling hopeful or
scared with each announcement of a new nutrition study, people could
turn to their index of food tale types and categorize the study. Let's give
it a try with a recent dietary scare!

> *Synthesized from seaweed. Identified as toxic to humans. Pronounced*
> *potentially unsafe for infants. Accused of causing digestive problems,*
> *chronic fatigue, diabetes, migraines, Alzheimer's, Parkinson's, heart dis-*
> *ease, and cancer.*

These identifying points signal a type of food tale with which we
are all too familiar: "unnatural substance causes multiple chronic illnesses." Within this subcategory, there's even a recurring plotline:
"toxic additive produced by processing seaweed." This is the story of
MSG, and it is unfolding again with another widely used substance
called carrageenan.

As a new dietary demon, carrageenan is tailor-made to terrify
health food enthusiasts. Employed primarily as an emulsifier, thicken-
ing agent, and a plant-based gelatin substitute, carrageenan is found in
dairy products, soy milk, almond milk, nutritional supplements, and
meal replacement shakes, many of which appear in the diets of health-
conscious eaters.

Tale types are particularly useful because they predict the structure
of any tale that fits the type. In other words, once we know the story
of MSG, the story of carrageenan should follow the same formulaic
plotline. Does it?

1. MSG was first vilified by a single group of scientists.
   The scare over carrageenan has been based on the work
   and activism of one scientist, Dr. Joanne Tobacman of
   the University of Illinois College of Medicine. At first

Tobacman focused on the potential role of carrageenan in causing breast cancer. The FDA and the European Scientific Committee on Food rejected the cancer hypothesis. She has now shifted her focus to connecting carrageenan with irritable bowel syndrome and diabetes.

2. Anti-MSG advocates succeeded in getting MSG removed from infant formula, despite any conclusive evidence supporting that decision. The same is true for carrageenan, which was banned from infant formula in Europe without a scientific basis. From the Food and Agriculture Organization of the United Nations and the World Health Organization in June 2014: *"The Committee concluded that the use of carrageenan in infant formula or formula for special medical purposes . . . is not of concern."*

3. Public pressure forced companies to remove MSG from their products. In August 2014, the "Food Babe" and her "Food Babe Army" pressured WhiteWave Foods, owners of Horizon Organic and Silk, into removing carrageenan from all of their products.

The story of carrageenan is just beginning, but the tale type tells us everything we need to know. (By the time you read this, the following predictions may already have come true.) Activists will call carrageenan unnatural. They will distinguish between "naturally occurring carrageenan" found in seaweed, and the unnatural synthesized carrageenan employed by Big Food. Celebrity doctors like Dr. Oz will hop on the bandwagon. As a good scapegoat, carrageenan will be linked to all the usual suspects: autism, Alzheimer's, ADHD, cancer, diabetes, and every chronic disease imaginable. Finally, scientists will spend untold hours and dollars trying to exonerate the additive. Their efforts will fail, and the myth of carrageenan toxicity will live on for decades, until it is finally eclipsed by another set of fairy tales.

Everything Does Not Cause (or Cure) Cancer

The truth about what we eat is unromantic. There are no dietary villains or miracle cures. There is no paradise past, no noble savage, no magic elixir, no one true diet. The demons are the gurus and fearmongers who make you sick with anxiety, identifying endless toxins and hidden killers, then offering advice that will save you from the nutritional hell they themselves created.

Since the gurus and fearmongers do not base their advice on sound, settled science, the world of food rules is confusing and cacophonous. Just think about the battle between vegetarians and meat eaters. The documentary *Forks Over Knives* contends that "most, if not all, of the degenerative diseases that afflict us can be controlled, or even reversed, by rejecting animal-based and processed foods." Citations of official studies abound. Pounds are dropped, lives are transformed. Dr. Oz says he "loved it and needs all of you to see it."

Strangely, Dr. Oz also endorses *Wheat Belly* and *Grain Brain*, books that argue the opposite of *Forks Over Knives*. While *Forks Over Knives* recommends eating whole grains as part of an ideal diet, *Wheat Belly* and *Grain Brain* strictly forbid these addictive toxins, which cause everything from obesity to Alzheimer's. David Perlmutter assures his readers that avoiding animal fat is downright dangerous, depriving our brains of the fat they desperately crave. (Hear an echo of "you are what you eat"? A brain made of animal fat requires animal fat to sustain itself.) Citations of official studies abound. Pounds are dropped, lives are transformed.

What to believe? Whom to believe? Should we eat meat or not? Lean meat or fatty meat? Does grilling create carcinogens? Does broccoli prevent cancer? Are artificial sweeteners safe? Can I drink from plastic bottles? Does running prevent heart disease?

The questions and conflicting answers just keep coming, and we keep listening. The silliness of identifying dietary demons and super-foods was documented in a 2013 systematic review published in the *American Journal of Clinical Nutrition*, titled "Is everything we eat associated with cancer?" The review found that 80 percent of common ingredients had been connected with cancer risk in published articles, with most of those reporting a statistically significant effect, either positive or negative. Analysis of the studies, however, showed that they usually highlighted "implausibly large effects, even though evidence is weak."

Put differently: whenever you read a headline about some new carcinogen or cancer-fighting superfood, it's probably not worth reading any further.

Whenever you read a headline about some new carcinogen or cancer-fighting superfood, it's probably not worth reading any further.

The unpleasant reality is we don't know what constitutes an "ideal" diet, and there may be no such thing. *Forks Over Knives*, *Grain Brain*, *Wheat Belly*, and Master Halewind's recipe for eternal youth—they just aren't worth your attention. What's left? Eat in moderation, drink in moderation, don't be sedentary. That's it. Veganism, fat-free, salt-free, sugar-free, gluten-free, Paleo, juicing, cleansing—these offer false promises built on myth and superstition, covered over with a layer of scientific rhetoric.

Myths Are Infectious

Nonsensical dietary advice isn't just false—it's dangerous. Worship of Nature, noble savages that climb trees to gather honey, the myth of paradise past—these fantasies slide too easily into condemnation of other modern medical innovations, which, unlike fad diets, are directly responsible for saving lives.

True, there's nothing wrong with people wearing toe shoes in imitation of their Paleolithic ancestors, and it's entertaining to watch the company making those toe shoes get sued for false advertising (as Vibram USA did in 2014, a lawsuit they settled for $3.75 million). No real harm will come to people who avoid salt and high-fructose corn syrup because they are "unnatural."

But it's not so funny when people avoid unnatural vaccines. Unfortunately, fear of modern medicine is a direct consequence of belief in common dietary myths. Just read the following passages from a 1922 herbal medicine pamphlet, which, aside from the racist language, could have been taken directly from a modern Paleolithic diet website or an anti-vaccine manifesto:

> Why use poisonous drugs when nature in her wisdom and beneficence has provided, in her great vegetable laboratories—the field and forests—relief for most of the ills of mankind?
>
> As a matter of fact, an honest doctor will admit that the latest medical science is not more uniformly successful in the treatment of many ills and maladies than the remedies discovered and used for centuries past by numerous tribes of Indians and other savage races. Again and again, in highly civilized nations we have seen whole communities exterminated—thousands of people slain by epidemics and plagues in spite of all that physicians could do.
>
> It is not easy to think of the Indians of North and South America, the black people of Africa and the islands of the sea and the yellow races of Asia as possessing scientific knowledge. Yet if these people had not found a cure for hundreds of their ailments, they must long since have disappeared from the earth. The answer is quite simple—Nature does the curing.

A search for "Paleo" and "vaccines" turns up numerous websites that reject vaccines by appealing to the myth of paradise past, noble savages, and natural healing. In "Why Vaccines Aren't Paleo," an article laden with impressive citations, Kelly Brogan, a Cornell-educated psychiatrist, implores her readers to "honor a wisdom in evolution" that inveighs against toxic modern food *and* toxic vaccinations. "Contrary to the claim that vaccines eliminate infection, they promote it," she says. Before modern food, our hearty, healthy ancestors were naturally resistant to disease—and Dr. Brogan promises that if we eat what they ate, we can be too.

She's not alone. Paleo guru and licensed acupuncturist Chris Kresser admits he decided not to vaccinate his nine-month-old daughter, choosing to rely on the resistance to disease conferred by eating like a Neanderthal. Sociologist Jennifer Reich of the University of Denver has studied mothers who refuse vaccines, and summarizes their attitude as follows:

> Mothers in my study describe their efforts to protect their children's health in ways they see as making vaccines unnecessary. They focus on organic foods, breastfeeding, health-promoting practices at home. . . . As experts on their own children, women saw their efforts as superior to the generic recommendations made by medical professionals who did not know their children.

Relying on the "natural" disease resistance conferred by organic foods and breast-feeding makes sense until there's an outbreak of measles, mumps, whooping cough, polio, or rubella. Try curing those with goji berries and buttered coffee. Everyday foods in reasonable amounts don't cause diseases—but toxic beliefs can.

You Are Not What You Eat

This is why it's so important to unmask nutrition myths. The paranoid false logic that motivates them seeps into other parts of our culture, poisoning whatever it touches. Look at how the myth of *you are what you eat* carries over into the metaphorical "consumption" of media, leading to the unfounded belief that viewing violent content causes people to become violent. Long before TV and video games, anxious parents and religious figures argued that violent comic books posed a grave moral danger to children. In 1948, psychiatrist Fredric Wertham legitimated their fears in a popular article for *Collier's Weekly*, "Horror in the Nursery." His studies of delinquent and disturbed children showed that comic books, with their "kicking and punching" and "wonderfully chesty girls," were a significant factor in every case. Ignoring Aristotle's theory that viewing violence might be cathartic, not inspirational, Wertham accused psychiatrists who defended comics of being "prima donnas" who sit on committees and fail to treat actual children. Those who did treat them, as he did, couldn't fail to recognize that the consumption of violent books and images created violent children.

Wertham's work contributed to a book burning later that year in Spencer, West Virginia, where 600 children made a comic-book bonfire, supervised by parents, teachers, and priests. The plausibility of the link between violent media and violent behavior inspired thousands of studies on television and video games, the vast majority of which would confirm what they set out to find. These, in turn, lent plausibility to popular arguments that blamed gun violence on TV and video games. Recent studies, however, have cast grave doubt on the connection, with psychologist Christopher Ferguson of Texas A&M leading the way in arguing that moral panic, not scholarly rigor, may have driven many of the findings against violent media. Attention to the implications of *you are what you eat* suggests that superstition gives this particular moral panic additional unwarranted credibility.

Paradise past. Noble savages. You are what you eat. Before you know it, we're neo-Puritan witch-hunters, monitoring media for the latest study confirming modernity is evil. Video games make children into monsters. Cell phones cause brain cancer. The Internet destroys our attention span. All the while, we forget to be grateful for what is without question the healthiest period in the history of humankind.

Eating in the Fourth Dimension

We are sick, for sure—sick with needless anxiety. The cure isn't in our food, it's in our minds. In truth, the only elimination diet most people should be trying is one that eliminates myths and superstitions about food.

I realize this may not be enough for people who want concrete advice on what they should be eating. Skepticism doesn't generate clear rules. There's no such thing as a sarcastic food pyramid. If you are genuinely interested in guidance, debunked food myths and dietary advice are not that helpful. A fundamental human need remains unsatisfied, the need to be told how to eat right—to eat righteously—and in so doing avoid disease and death. Into this void step the Daoist monks, the authors of Leviticus, the government officials, the overconfident scientists, the neo-Puritan nutritionists, the hard-bodied Paleo Diet gurus, the TV doctors, your Facebook feed. We want to know—*need to know*—WHAT TO EAT!

Although there are drastic differences between the regimens these gurus recommend, they all focus on three primary dimensions of food. *Category*: fruit or vegetable, carb or protein. *Quality*: the effect of the food on one's overall physical well-being. *Quantity*: the amount of food being consumed. Diets universally involve rules about these three dimensions, from Weight Watchers to low carb to vegetarian to Paleo. Most people can't imagine healthy eating in any other way.

> **The only elimination diet most people should be trying is one that eliminates myths and superstitions about food.**

Yet what if that's the biggest dietary mistake our culture is making? As Paul Rozin points out, the French have lower rates of heart disease and are leaner than their American counterparts—and they are far *less* obsessed with the healthfulness of what they eat. Numerous studies suggest that although some people successfully lose weight by dieting, in the majority of cases *dieting results in more weight gain than doing nothing at all*. One study of Finnish twins found that, independent of genetics, dieting predicted a three- to five-times *greater* likelihood of obesity! Remember: for every enthusiastic public testimonial about a diet book resulting in miraculous weight loss, there are far more silent failures that led to weight gain and binge-eating disorders.

Meanwhile, our Fitbit step-trackers, calorie counting, and obsession with nutritional value are ruining culinary culture. In the 1940s, the philosophers Max Horkheimer and Theodor Adorno warned about people who "converted the stroll into exercise and food into calories." Those who do that, they said, lose their souls and turn life "into a chemical process." Their description of calorie-counters and health nuts—the Food Babe Army and the elimination dieters, Dr. Oz and nutrition gurus—is terrifyingly accurate: "They are interested in illness, anticipating their fellow diner's death in what he eats, their interest being only thinly rationalized by concern for his health." Dietary myths and superstitions are turning people into latter-day food crusaders, not unlike the European crusaders who hunted invented infidels in order to give their own lives meaning—and, in the case of their leaders, make a few bucks in the process.

Some are completely lost to this new, empty religion. Sadly, I can offer them no real hope. But if you are like me, you are sick of feeling like every dietary choice you make is a life-and-death decision. You want to relax about food. You don't want to feel guilty about enjoying cuisine. Yet you see these dietary evangelists and wonder, *What if they're right?* If that's how you feel, I invite you to break free of anxiety, absurd laws, and empty promises with a simple technique that I have personally employed with great success: *eating in the fourth dimension.*

When you eat in the fourth dimension, there are no rules about category, quality, and quantity of food. Eating in the fourth dimension is compatible with all recipes from every culinary culture. No foods are forbidden. You don't have to shop organic or count calories. The only aspect of your food that matters is *time*: the time you spend preparing it and the time you spend consuming it.

So let me borrow from the authors of *Grain Brain* and *Wheat Belly* and ask you to conduct an experiment. For one month, try eating in the fourth dimension. There are only two rules:

1. Whenever you eat, your time must be undivided. No eating while driving, or walking, or watching a movie, or watching a sporting event. This isn't some weird "no talking while eating" rule—of course you can have family meals or meals with friends. Don't overthink it. The idea is that for one month, you *set aside time to eat, rather than eating during time you've set aside for something else.*

2. Make sure that four dinners a week take at least thirty minutes to prepare and twenty minutes to eat. Don't worry about what or how much you're eating. Choose your recipes without any consideration of calories, salt, fat, gluten, or sugar. Just prepare your food with care and eat it slowly, seated at a table.

As for the rest of your meals—it doesn't matter. Eat whatever you want. Go out for beer and pizza. Have a store-bought smoothie and a dough-nut for breakfast. As long as you follow both rules, you are eating in the fourth dimension.

There's actually a third rule, but it has nothing to do with your food. Like any good diet plan, eating in the fourth dimension involves a detox. During your trial month, eliminate *all reading about nutrition or health*. Does the *New York Times* have an article about gluten? Don't read it. Did someone post a scary story about carrageenan and autism on Facebook? Just keep scrolling. Tempted to check out the nutrition label on the can of chicken broth you're using to make your soup? Stop! Don't break the detox. It's just thirty days. You can do it. (If this sounds tough to you, maybe you are a health information "addict.")

My prediction is that by the end of the month you'll feel much, much better, mentally and physically. Eating in the fourth dimension means you don't have to worry about the endless contradictory studies, the miracle foods and dietary demons. After a few weeks, arguments about which diet is best will start looking like debates about how many angels can dance on the head of a pin. Other people's food fears will reveal themselves

Food will be food, and when that happens, its true powers will be revealed.

as religious taboos. Your guilt and anxiety will disappear, as you enjoy the meal you prepared for yourself, your friends, or your family. You will "boost your immunity" to lies and pseudoscience, and you will face the uncertainties of life and health without depending on panaceas and fairy tales. Food will no longer be medicine or poison, good or evil. It won't cause or prevent disease, cut life short or extend it. Food will be food, and when that happens, its true powers will be revealed.

I guarantee it.

Bonus Miracle Diet Plan!

Needless to say, I don't want any of my readers to be disappointed. If, after a month, you aren't satisfied with eating in the fourth dimension, I have developed an alternative diet plan that's sure to please.

You see, during the course of researching this book, something amazing happened: *I discovered the secret truth about modern illnesses and developed the first diet that will protect against them while simultaneously extending your life.*

Obesity, Alzheimer's, cancer, ADHD, autism, heart disease, chronic fatigue syndrome: all these and more can be avoided, provided you eat correctly. And it's easy! With one simple change to your eating habits, you will be able to prevent or reverse chronic disease and ensure you live to a ripe old age.

What? Aren't I contradicting myself? Hasn't this whole book been about debunking just these kinds of claims?

It may seem that way at first, but before you come to any conclusions, please read on. You'll see that unlike other diets, my diet plan is 100 percent supported by science. I solve riddles that no other diet has the courage to address. And I reveal the truth that nutritionists, obesity doctors, and diet gurus don't want you to know, because if you did, *they'd be out of a job.*

So if eating in the fourth dimension hasn't healed you, try my UNpacked Diet.™ And, don't forget to keep reading to see how it was developed. What do you have to lose besides your brain fog and those extra pounds?

The UNpacked Diet™

UNpack your pounds. UNpack your potential. UNpack your food.

Finally: a scientifically proven revolution in healthy eating!

- Learn why what you eat isn't the problem.

- Learn why nutritionists and scientists always disagree about which foods are bad and which foods are good.

- Stop listening to the hype and start living the truth.

- Embrace the UNpacked Diet™ . . . and say goodbye to fad diets forever!

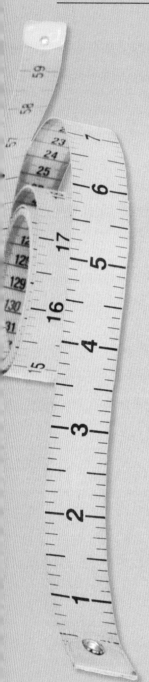

UNpacked 9-Day Detox

Here's my promise: With JUST 9 days on the UNpacked Diet, you'll be jump-started on the path to health. Some people, including doctors, don't think you can radically transform your health in a few days, but I do. Why? Because I've seen it happen with my own eyes. Just follow my proven program, and in 9 days not only can you lose up to 9 pounds, but you can also prevent or reverse chronic health problems including diabetes, asthma, joint pain, digestive problems, auto-immune disease, headaches, brain fog, allergies, acne, eczema, and even sexual dysfunction.

Step One: Be Honest With Yourself

Weigh yourself. Measure your waistline. Then think back to the last time you felt completely rested and fully energized. Now, ask yourself: Is this the real you, or is someone different—leaner, smarter, happier, better—hidden inside, trying to escape? Are you ready to help?

Step Two: Read the UNpacked Diet

Find out what's keeping you from becoming your true self. You'll be shocked, you'll be angry, and you'll be em-powered to make the changes that will start you on the road to health. Best of all—you'll be able to eat every single food you love: carbs, fats, salt, sugar, wheat, meat, dairy. Unlike other diets, when you UNpack, you really don't have to give up anything.

Step Three: 9-Day Detox

For just nine days, UNpack your diet. Then go back to step one. Weigh yourself. Measure your waistline. Then think back to the last time you felt completely rested and fully energized. Now, ask yourself: Have you started UNpacking the pounds, like so many other people have? Have you started UNpacking your potential?

Of course you have! So make the UNpacked Diet a lifestyle, not just a diet!

Why Us, Why Now?

Think back to the traditional meals your great-grandmother and grandmother prepared: huge bowls of mashed potatoes, giant beef roasts, pale bread rolls slathered in butter, fresh-baked pies with flaky lard crusts. Your parents probably have fond memories of chasing after the ice cream truck every day of summer. And we have beautiful vintage Coca-Cola ads to remind us of a time when kids guiltlessly drank a bottle of Coke whenever the days were hot.

How did they get away with eating like that, when today the same types of foods are said to cause chronic disease?

Conventional wisdom tells us that unhealthy eating habits cause the obesity, hypertension, heart disease, stroke, and diabetes that plague our modern world. New research shows that diet can also cause psychological conditions like ADHD, Alzheimer's, schizophrenia, and autism.

But which foods are the problem? Scientists and diet gurus "whiplash" us back and forth on the culprits—from salt to sugar to fat to gluten. Do you trust the Paleolithic crowd? That means red meat is fine and whole grains are dangerous. Do you trust our government? Then whole grains are a must, and red meat will give you cancer and heart disease. Mainstream nutritionists will tell you it's all about energy balance—just eat fewer calories than you burn. But if you're among those who have tried diet and exercise, you *know* there's more to the story.

Looking to traditional cultures for our optimal diet raises even more questions. We know that African Masai tribes stay disease-free on a diet of raw milk and meat.[1] Yet we attribute the great health of the ancient Chinese to their nearly vegetarian diet.[2] The Yanomamo Indians of Brazil thrive on a salt-free diet, whereas the Japanese (one of the healthiest modern cultures with virtually no heart disease) eat the highest-sodium diet in the world.[3,4]

Could it be that conventional wisdom is only *partially* right?

There is something wrong with our diet. Of course there is! Look at the skyrocketing rates of obesity, chronic disease, cancer, and mental illness.

But here's the shocking truth: the *type* of food we eat isn't the problem.

The *only* thing everyone agrees on is that sick, obese America eats too much processed and packaged food. According to a *New York Times* report, Americans eat 31 percent more packaged food than fresh food. We eat more packaged food than almost any other country. But don't jump to conclusions about what's in those packages. Nearly 40 percent of packaged-food consumption in America comes from dairy, especially heart-healthy yogurt and skim milk. Only 6 percent of our packaged-food consumption comes from those

---

[1] Friedrich-Schiller-Universität Jena, "Nomadic People's Good Health Baffles Scientists," ScienceDaily, May 18, 2010.

[2] Keith Akers, A Vegetarian Sourcebook: The Nutrition, Ecology, and Ethics of a Vegetarian Diet, (Vegetarian Press, 1983).

[3] William J. Oliver, Edwin L. Cohen, and James V. Neel, "Blood Pressure, Sodium Intake, and Sodium Related Hormones in the Yanomamo Indians, a 'No-Salt' Culture," Circulation 52.1 (1975): 146–51.

[4] Taichi Shimazu, et al., "Dietary Patterns and Cardiovascular Disease Mortality in Japan: A Prospective Cohort Study," International Journal of Epidemiology 36.3 (2007): 600–609.

snacks and candy we associate with weight gain and disease.[5]

In fact, as food manufacturers and fast-food chains produce "healthier" options, including low-fat meals, cultured dairy, whole grain breads, and preprepared salads, our health continues to decline. It seems like the harder we try and the more we know, the worse things get.

So let's ask again: What has *really* changed since the healthier generations of our past? What do they and the Yanomamo and the Masai all have in common?

When I think of my 95-year-old grandmother, I always think of a glass jar. In fact, her kitchen was filled with them. At the end of the summer, she would stuff jars with fruits and vegetables to preserve and eat all year long.

Today, glass is infrequently used to store food, and for one simple reason: Big Food wants to keep things cheap. Gone is Grandmother's pantry. Kitchens are now filled with plastics, metals, and heavily bleached and processed papers. Many people have never even seen a traditional burlap sack. Instead, our rice and grains are sealed into plastic bags. Milk, which once came delivered fresh in glass jugs, sits for days in plastic containers or plastic-lined cartons. Our grandparents brought fresh produce home in crates and cartons. We get our fruits and veggies precut, conveniently shrink-wrapped in plastic and Styrofoam.

Our Paleolithic ancestors ate a wide variety of diets depending on where they lived.[6] But none of them

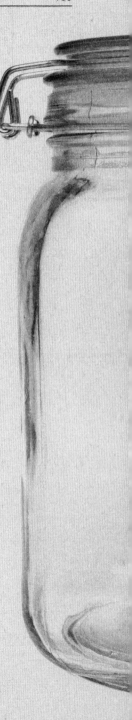

---

[5] www.nytimes.com/imagepates/2010/04/04/business/04metrics_g.html.

[6] Marlene Zuk, *Paleofantasy: What Evolution Really Tells Us about Sex, Diet, and How We Live* (New York: W. W. Norton & Company, 2013).

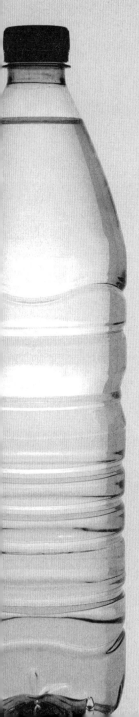

shopped at grocery stores. They found their food in Nature, wrapped in Nature's packaging of peels and husks. Food today is a different story. Wherever it is found, from gas station mini-marts to giant Walmarts, it almost always comes packaged. And even when it doesn't, we place it in plastic bags ourselves before taking it home to feed our families.

If we are willing to ignore old ways of thinking about food, the answer to our dietary problems is obvious. The whiplash goes away when we stop trying to figure which *type* of food is the dietary villain, or which new fad diet will help us lose weight and get rid of chronic disease. Science can't tell us which diet is right because there *isn't* a right diet!

Here's what science can tell us, and it's what all those whiplashing diet gurus and nutritionists don't want you know, because they'd be out of a job. The most common supermarket and fast-food materials—plastic, aluminum, tin, even recycled paper—contain dangerous chemicals and heavy metals that fatten us up and destroy our health.

The real villain is in the packaging.

Plastics Are Not Fantastic

The dangers of plastics are no surprise to scientists, who have been studying their negative health effects for decades. Researchers and health officials have voiced concerns about "nanoplastics" (small plastic particles) that get into our food by "leaching" or "migration." Although Big Chem and Big Food have done their best to suppress this information, numerous studies prove the health risks are enormous.

Unlike low carb vs. low fat, there is no debate about the dangers of these modern food storage materials.

You may have heard about the most notorious of these plastics, BPA. Polycarbonate plastics (containing BPA) are extremely common in US food packaging. In 2004, the CDC found traces of BPA in nearly all the urine samples it collected (93 percent of adults), and scientists predict that today the number would be over 99 percent.[7] The source of this BPA is primarily our diets.[8]

The dangers of this poisonous endocrine disrupter are almost too numerous to list. BPA mimics estrogen and has been shown to grow breast cancer cells.[9] Exposure to BPA early in life leads to precancerous changes in the prostate and mammary glands, altered brain development, lower sperm counts, chromosomal abnormalities in eggs, obesity, and insulin resistance.[10] Prenatal exposure to BPA correlates with breast cancer later in life, a fact so alarming that the Breast Cancer Fund urges people to avoid *all BPA plastics*.[11] They also recommend eliminating canned food, since BPA is commonly used in can lining.[12]

---

[7] Antonia M. Calafat, et al., "Exposure of the US population to Bisphenol A and 4-Tertiary-Octylphenol: 2003–2004," *Environmental Health Perspectives* (2008): 39–44.

[8] L Trasande, TM Attina, and J Blustein, "Association between Urinary Bisphenol A Concentration and Obesity Prevalence in Children and Adolescents," *JAMA* 308 (2012): 1113–21.

[9] Endocrine Society, "BPA Stimulates Growth of an Advanced Subtype of Human Breast Cancer Cells Called Inflammatory Breast Cancer," ScienceDaily, June 23, 2014.

[10] www.medicalnewstoday.com/articles/243626.php.

[11] Endocrine Society, "BPA Exposure in Utero May Increase Predisposition to Breast Cancer," ScienceDaily, October 3, 2011.

[12] www.breastcancerfund.org/reduce-your-risk/tips/eat-live-better.

Just think about the implications for so-called healthy eaters. An independent, nonindustry Breast Cancer Fund study looked at more than 300 products and found BPA levels were highest in some of the "healthiest" low-calorie foods such as canned vegetables, soup, and lite coconut milk.[13] That puts those who think they are making smart food choices at the highest risk.

Thankfully, BPA buildup may be reversible. In 2011, the Breast Cancer Fund, in conjunction with the Silent Spring Institute, put a BPA detox diet to the test. Their study, published in *Environmental Health Perspectives* (a prestigious journal overseen by the National Institute of Health), tested families who adopted a diet that eliminated all packaged foods. By the end of the study, BPA levels had dropped by an astonishing 60 percent![14]

---

[13] Breast Cancer Fund (2010), What Labels Don't Tell Us: Getting BPA out of Our Food and Our Bodies, www.breastcancerfund.org/assets/pdfs/publications/what-labels-dont-tell-us-1.pdf.

[14] Ruthann A. Rudel, et al., "Food Packaging and Bisphenol A and Bis (2-Ethyhexyl) Phthalate Exposure: Findings from a Dietary Intervention," *Environmental Health Perspectives* 119.7 (2011): 914–20.

WOULD YOU LIKE YOUR RECEIPT? Cash register receipts are coated with BPA, which absorbs into the skin. If you are highly BPA-sensitive, consider shopping with gloves or declining the receipt.

Considered toxic in Canada and outlawed across the European Union, it's amazing that BPA is still used at all. Although the FDA has finally banned BPA from baby bottles, Big Food and Big Chem continue to fight against further regulation. Instead, they encourage us to focus on "healthy foods," cranking out low-cal, low-fat product lines that depend on the cheap packaging that's at the heart of our nation's health problems.

Frighteningly, BPA is just the tip of the iceberg. Another 2011 study from *Environmental Health Perspectives* tested 500 chemical containers and found that nearly all of them, even those previously considered safe, release estrogen-mimicking chemicals. BPA-free products, including baby bottles, actually release synthetic estrogens that are *more potent than BPA!*[15] Stuart Yaniger, one of the lead authors of the study, put it bluntly: "Baby bottles, plastic bags, plastic wrap, clamshell food containers, stand-up pouches: Just about anything you can think of that's made of plastic that food or beverages are wrapped up in, we found this activity. It was shocking to us."[16]

---

[15] *Environmental Health Perspectives* 119 (2011): 989–96. dx.doi.org/10.1289/ehp.1003220. [online March 2, 2011]

[16] www.chriskresser.com/how-plastic-food-containers-could-be-making-you-fat-infertile-and-sick.

Yaniger's warning about plastic wrap is particularly important. Plastic wraps are known to contain an extremely dangerous endocrine disrupter called DEHA (*diethyl hexyl adipate*). Panicked industry groups continue to deny its toxicity, but unbiased researchers keep linking DEHA to liver tumors, asthma, and cancer.[17] Consumers Union research confirmed that food wrapped in plastic, like deli cheeses, had DEHA levels exceeding levels considered safe in Europe.[18] You wouldn't wrap your food in a poison-soaked cloth, but that's exactly what you're doing when you wrap your food in plastic contaminated with DEHA.

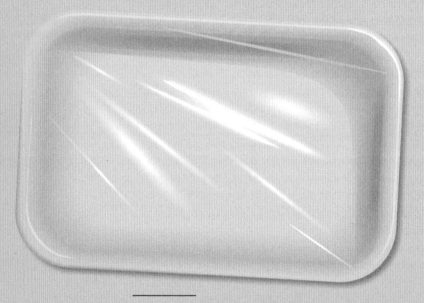

[17] www.center4research.org/healthy-living-prevention/products-with-health-risks/plastic-wrap-and-plastic-food-containers-are-they-safe.

[18] www.consumersunion.org/news/report-to-the-fda-regarding-plastic-packaging.

As use of plastic increases, so do rates of mental disorders like ADHD and autism.[19] While the two seem intuitively unrelated, scientists see a connection. Irva Hertz-Picciotto, chief of the Division of Environmental and Occupational Health at UC Davis, believes that because plastic packaging interferes with the body's natural hormonal system, it could "play a role in autism or other neurodevelopmental disorders." Other doctors suspect plastic packaging may disrupt thyroid hormone, which is critical for brain development. Thyroid dysfunction is particularly common in children with autism.[20]

And those migraines? They aren't just in your head. According to the Mayo Clinic, plastics may be responsible for your migraine. The hormones estrogen and progesterone play key roles in regulating menstruation and pregnancy, which affect headache-causing chemicals in the brain.[21] Steady estrogen levels improve headaches, but altered levels make them worse. A University of Kansas study found that hormone-disrupting plastics caused migraine symptoms, including light and sound sensitivity.[22] Chemicals in plastic food packaging have also been linked to heart disease,[23] adult

[19] www.articles.mercola.com/sites/articles/archive/2014/04/02/environmental-toxin-exposure.aspx.

[20] www.thechart.blogs.cnn.com/2011/06/07/scientists-warn-of-chemical-autism-link.

[21] www.mayoclinic.org/diseases-conditions/chronic-daily-headaches/in-depth/headaches/art-20046729.

[22] NEJ Berman, E Gregory, KE McCarson et al., "Exposure to Bisphenol A Exacerbates Migraine-Like Behaviors in a Multibehavior Model of Rat Migraine," Toxicological Sciences 137.2 (2014): 416–27.

[23] Naomi Lubick, "Cardiovascular Health: Exploring a Potential Link between BPA and Heart Disease," Environmental Health Perspectives 118.3 (2010): A116.

onset diabetes,[24] high blood pressure,[25] early puberty,[26] allergies,[27] asthma,[28] anxiety,[29] unattractiveness,[30] erectile dysfunction,[31] depression,[32] schizophrenia,[33] and Alzheimer's.[34]

So plastics make us sick—but do they also make us fat? The answer is clear. Scientists have known for over a decade that plastics cause obesity in rats, and recently found that the link extends to humans. In the 2012 Smithsonian.com article "Is the Can Worse Than the Soda?," author Joseph Stromberg cites the first

[24] Ben Harder, "Diabetes from a Plastic?: Estrogen Mimic Provokes Insulin Resistance," Science News 169.3 (2006): 36–37.

[25] Leonardo Trasande, et al., "Urinary Phthalates Are Associated with Higher Blood Pressure in Childhood," Journal of Pediatrics 163.3 (2013): 747–53.

[26] Jonathan R. Roy, Sanjoy Chakraborty, and Tandra R. Chakraborty, "Estrogen-Like Endocrine Disrupting Chemicals Affecting Puberty in Humans: A Review," Medical Science Monitor 15.6 (2009): 137–45.

[27] Datis Kharrazian, "The Potential Roles of Bisphenol A (BPA) Pathogenesis in Autoimmunity," Autoimmune Diseases, vol. 2014, Article ID 743616, 12 pages, 2014. doi:10.1155/2014/743616.

[28] Carl-Gustaf Bornehag, et al., "The Association between Asthma and Allergic Symptoms in Children and Phthalates in House Dust: A Nested Case-Control Study," Environmental Health Perspectives (2004): 1393–97.

[29] Bryce C. Ryan, and John G. Vandenbergh, "Developmental Exposure to Environmental Estrogens Alters Anxiety and Spatial Memory in Female Mice." Hormones and Behavior 50.1 (2006): 85–93.

[30] Lisa A. M. Galea, and Cindy K. Barha, "Maternal Bisphenol A (BPA) Decreases Attractiveness of Male Offspring," Proceedings of the National Academy of Sciences 108.28 (2011): 11305–6.

[31] De-Kun Li, et al., "Relationship between Urine Bisphenol-A Level and Declining Male Sexual Function," Journal of Andrology 31.5 (2010): 500–506.

[32] www.rodalenews.com/multiple-chemical-sensitivity.

[33] James S. Brown, "Effects of Bisphenol-A and Other Endocrine Disruptors Compared with Abnormalities of Schizophrenia: An Endocrine-Disruption Theory of Schizophrenia," Schizophrenia Bulletin 35.1 (2009): 256–78.

[34] Wei Sun, et al., "Perinatal Exposure to Di-(2-Ethylhexyl)-Phthalate Leads to Cognitive Dysfunction and Phospho-Tau Level Increase in Aged Rats," Environmental Toxicology (2012).

large-scale study (with a sample of around 3,000 children) to find a significant link between BPA and obesity. Stromberg notes the study "hints at the surprisingly complex root causes of obesity, once thought to simply reflect an imbalance between caloric intake and exercise."[35] A later study in the journal *Pediatrics* looked at 3,300 children ages six to eighteen and found that those with high BPA levels tended to have "excessive amounts of body fat and unusually expanded waistlines."[36] A 2013 study by Kaiser Permanente found that girls with higher levels of BPA were *five times more likely to be overweight.*[37] Several studies have linked plastics to expanded waistlines and insulin resistance. One 2013 study in *Environmental Health Perspectives* found plastic exposure put African American children especially at risk for obesity. The authors reported that every unit increase of nanoplastics in their urine meant a 21 percent higher chance the child would be overweight and 22 percent higher chance the child would be obese.[38]

It is no coincidence that when plastic use took off, we started packing on the pounds.

Styrofoam: A Heated Debate

Polystyrene, familiar to most of us as Styrofoam, is technically a type of plastic. It is commonly used for drinking cups, fast-food packaging, egg cartons, and takeout

---

[35] www.smithsonianmag.com/ist/?next=/science-nature/is-the-can-worse-than-the-soda-study-finds-correlation-between-bpa-and-obesity-40894828.

[36] Donna S. Eng, et al., "Bisphenol A and Chronic Disease Risk Factors in US Children," *Pediatrics* 132.3 (2013): e637–e645.

[37] De-Kun Li, Maohua Miao, ZhiJun Zhou, Chunhua Wu, Huijing Shi, Xiaoqin Liu, Siqi Wang, and Wei Yuan, "Urine Bisphenol-A Level in Relation to Obesity and Overweight in School-Age Children," *PLoS ONE*, 2013; 8 (6): e65399 DOI: 10.1371/journal.pone.0065399.

[38] Leonardo Trasande, et al., "Race/Ethnicity-Specific Associations of Urinary Phthalates with Childhood Body Mass in a Nationally Representative Sample," *Environmental Health Perspectives* 121.4 (2013): 501–506.

boxes. Although you find it everywhere, polystyrene foam contains styrene, which is a known carcinogen. A study of more than 12,000 male workers in a styrene polymer factory found styrene-exposed workers had an increased risk of leukemia and non-Hodgkin's lymphoma. The digestive system seems particularly susceptible to harm from styrene, as researchers also found higher rates of esophageal cancer in Caucasians and stomach cancer in blacks. Black workers exposed to styrene also had higher rates of heart disease.[39] Other observed health risks from styrene exposure include irritation of the skin, eyes, upper respiratory tract, and gastrointestinal problems.[40] That's not to mention "styrene sickness," a condition characterized by headaches, fatigue, brain fog, and depression.[41]

It is well documented that hot liquids cause Styrofoam to melt and break down. Health authorities say to never heat Styrofoam cups in the microwave, and warn against using them with warm beverages.[42] Yet Big Food continues to use polystyrene for their hot beverages and soups, and we keep drinking their products. One of the worst offenders is Dunkin' Donuts, which uses about 1 billion Styrofoam cups each year. There have been several petitions and a Facebook group dedicated to changing Dunkin' Donuts' packaging, but so far the company has resisted.[43] All along you've been wary of those trans-fat-filled doughnuts, when your Styrofoam

---

[39] Genevieve M. Matanoski, Carlos Santos-Burgoa, and Linda Schwartz, "Mortality of a Cohort of Workers in the Styrene-Butadiene Polymer Manufacturing Industry (1943–1982)," *Environmental Health Perspectives* 86 (1990): 107.

[40] www.earthresource.org/campaigns/capp/capp-styrofoam.html.

[41] www.rodalenews.com/coffee-and-styrofoam-cups.

[42] www.ewg.org/research/healthy-home-tips/tip-3-pick-plastics-carefully.

[43] www.facebook.com/pages/Encouraging-Dunkin-Donuts-to-stop-using-1-Billion-styrofoam-cups-a-year/199731989943.

KNOW YOUR PAPER. A paper cup can be a great safe alternative when you're on the go and forget your mug. But not all paper is created equal. Recycled paper in cereal boxes has been shown to cause cancer. Chlorine-bleached paper tea bags contain dioxin, a known carcinogen that can seep into your hot liquid.

coffee cup is the real killer. Can you believe it? Your Dunkin' coffee is worse than your Dunkin' Donut. Remember: *America* dies *on Dunkin'*!

But it turns out coffee is just a drop in the (plastic) bucket. Our greatest source of chemical disrupters comes from bottled water. Americans consume more than 9 billion gallons of bottled water a year, and rates are rising fast.[44] Although they don't look like Styrofoam, water bottles are made from polystyrene plastic. A 2006 study found high levels of styrene in brand-new bottled water samples. The levels increased over time as the bottled water sat on the shelf. When the bottles were heated, the levels were even higher, but even in fresh, cold water, the results were alarming![45] A later study published in the journal *Environmental Science and Pollution Research* confirmed that there were endocrine-disrupting chemicals in all the bottled water samples tested.[46]

---

[44] "Smaller categories still saw growth as the U.S. liquid refreshment beverage market shrunk by 2.0 percent in 2008, Beverage Marketing Corporation reports," press release, Beverage Marketing Corporation, March 30, 2009.

[45] Maqbool Ahmad and Ahmad S. Bajahlan, "Leaching of Styrene and Other Aromatic Compounds in Drinking Water from PS Bottles," *Journal of Environmental Sciences* 19.4 (2007): 421–26.

[46] Martin Wagner and Jörg Oehlmann, "Endocrine Disruptors in Bottled Mineral Water: Total Estrogenic Burden and Migration from Plastic Bottles," *Environmental Science and Pollution Research* 16.3 (2009): 278–86.

The following chart tracks bottled water consumption, and the curve almost exactly matches the growth of our obesity epidemic! Dietitians emphasize that drinking plenty of water is key to weight loss. Yet it's clear that drinking from bottles causes more than increased water weight.

As many of us strive to be healthy and hydrate, we find ourselves getting fatter and sicker. We drink our coffee black, without sugar or creamer, but that doesn't seem to help. We eat less at dinner and take the rest home in a takeout container, hoping to reduce our waistlines by reducing the size of our meals. But the sad truth is that all this focus on food is distracting us from the scientifically proven cause of our problems.

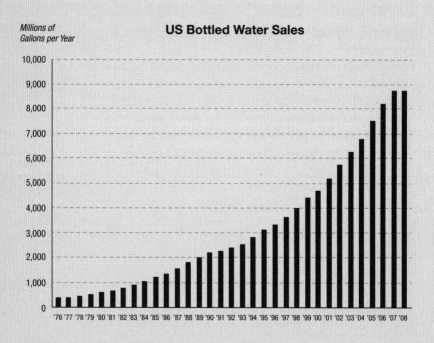

Millions of Gallons per Year

US Bottled Water Sales

Data from the US Department of Agriculture, Economic Research Service, and the Beverage Marketing Corporation.

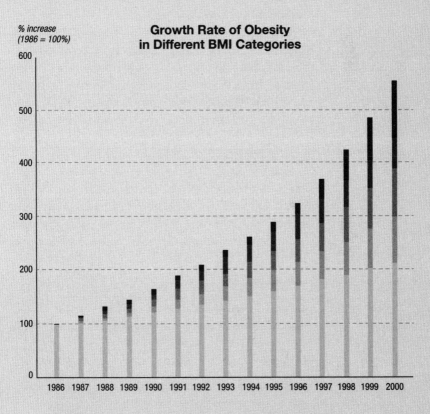

% increase
(1986 = 100%)

**Growth Rate of Obesity
in Different BMI Categories**

Source: R. Sturm, "Increases in clinically severe obesity in the
United States,1986–2000," *Arch. Intern. Med.* 163 (2003): 2146–49.

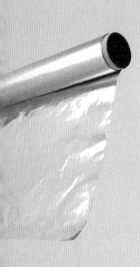

Aluminum Foiled

You might think that aluminum foil is a safe alternative for wrapping up home-cooked leftovers, but that's not true. One of the most dangerous metals lurking in our homes is aluminum.

Aluminum packaging wasn't in use until the twentieth century and is becoming increasingly popular. Global aluminum production today exceeds all metals except iron.[47] Although everyone has some amount of aluminum in the body, it provides no benefit or function. Aluminum accumulation, however, can be toxic. Aluminum has long been understood as a contributor to Alzheimer's disease, and numerous studies have confirmed the connection.[48] Scientists have found aluminum at the core of brain plaques associated with Alzheimer's.[49] But the dangers go beyond that well-known association. Aluminum exposure has been linked to everything from breast cancer to osteoporosis.[50,51] In fact, aluminum has been found to negatively inhibit more than 200 biological functions.[52]

Just as plastic leaches chemicals, research has shown that hazardous metals migrate into food when it is in contact with aluminum. So much aluminum gets into our food that the country of Oman banned cooking with it in 2010 and restricts hot food contact to the shiny side only.[53] A 1996 Italian study first brought

---

[47] www.commodities-now.com/news/metals-and-mining/612-world-metal-production-surges.html.

[48] www.whfoods.com/genpage.php?tname=newtip&dbid=8.

[49] www.doctoroz.com/article/your-brain-protection-plan.

[50] P. D. Darbre, "Underarm Cosmetics Are a Cause of Breast Cancer," *European Journal of Cancer Prevention* 10.5 (2001): 389–94.

[51] Bengt Mjöberg, et al., "Aluminum, Alzheimer's Disease and Bone Fragility." *Acta Orthopaedica* 68.6 (1997): 511–14.

[52] Masahiro Kawahara and Midori Kato-Negishi, "Link between Aluminum and the Pathogenesis of Alzheimer's Disease: The Integration of the Aluminum and Amyloid Cascade Hypotheses," *International Journal of Alzheimer's Disease* (2011).

[53] www.thenational.ae/news/uae-news/aluminium-foil-linked-to-osteoporosis-and-alzheimers.

> **TIN CANS: THE SAFER ALTERNATIVE?** Tin and aluminum are both popular canning materials. Tin exposure can cause skin and eye irritation, as well as neurological problems. And once a tin can is opened and the lining exposed to oxygen, corrosion occurs rapidly, releasing even more tin into your food.

alarm when it found 2–6 milligrams of aluminum transferred into food from foil, cookware, and utensils.[54] Follow-up studies have found even higher levels. A 2011 study in the *International Journal of Electrochemical Science* found that levels of aluminum were in toxic amounts well above the WHO safe limits in foods after they were cooked, reheated, or even simply cooled in aluminum foil. This effect was amplified by acidity—a point we will return to in a moment.[55]

Recently, scientists have directed their attention to the link between aluminum and obesity. Along with BPA in soda can liners, aluminum also helps pack on the pounds. High levels of aluminum in the body have been linked to iron deficiency, disproportionately common in those with obesity.[56] Biochemists in a 2007 report found that aluminum-induced mitochondrial dysfunction leads to obesity.[57]

---

[54] L. Gramiccioni, et al., "Aluminium Levels in Italian Diets and in Selected Foods from Aluminium Utensils." *Food Additives & Contaminants* 13.7 (1996): 767–74.

[55] F. S. Mohammad, E. A. H. Al Zubaidy, and G. Bassion, "Effect of Aluminum Leaching Process of Cooking Wares on Food," *International Journal of Electrochemical Science* 6.1 (2011): 222–230.

[56] Sungwon Han, et al., "How Aluminum, an Intracellular ROS Generator Promotes Hepatic and Neurological Diseases: The Metabolic Tale," *Cell Biology and Toxicology* 29.2 (2013): 75–84.

[57] Ryan Mailloux, Joseph Lemire, and Vasu Appanna, "Aluminum-Induced Mitochondrial Dysfunction Leads to Lipid Accumulation in Human Hepatocytes: A Link to Obesity," *Cellular Physiology and Biochemistry* 20.5 (2008): 627–38.

All this might help explain why diet sodas have been found to contribute to weight gain, a mystery that no nutrition experts can solve.[58] Remember how acidity amplifies the aluminum-leaching effect? A highly acidic zero-calorie beverage will still leach aluminum at a high rate. If you want to lose weight, you might be better off drinking a milk shake from a glass than a can of diet soda.

Frighteningly, research has also connected aluminum to learning disabilities and autism. As early as 2009, renowned neurosurgeon Russell Blaylock was examining how aluminum creates changes in the brain.[59] In a 2012 review titled "Empirical Data Confirm Autism Symptoms Related to Aluminum and Acetaminophen Exposure," the authors note that mentions of autism "increased steadily at the end of the last century, during a period when mercury was being phased out, while aluminum adjuvant burden was being increased." In the report, they link aluminum-containing vaccines to a significant rise in "cellulitis, seizure, depression, fatigue, pain and death."[60] In an article titled "Aluminum Toxicity in Mitochondrial Dysfunction and ASD," authors Nancy Mullan, MD, and Amy Yasko, PhD, AMD, FAAIM note the "intense interest and discussion surrounding the high incidence of mitochondrial disease

---

[58] Susan E. Swithers, "Artificial Sweeteners Produce the Counterintuitive Effect of Inducing Metabolic Derangements," *Trends in Endocrinology & Metabolism* 24.9 (2013): 431–41.

[59] Russell L. Blaylock, "A Possible Central Mechanism in Autism Spectrum Disorders, Part 3: The Role of Excitotoxin Food Additives and the Synergistic Effects of Other Environmental Toxins," *Alternative Therapies in Health and Medicine* 15.2 (2008): 56–60.

[60] Stephanie Seneff, Robert M. Davidson, and Jingjing Liu, "Empirical Data Confirm Autism Symptoms Related to Aluminum and Acetaminophen Exposure," *Entropy* 14.11 (2012): 2227–53.

and/or dysfunction in children with autism spectrum disorders." As there is no genetic cause of this dysfunction, attention is "turning away from genetics toward the environment."[61] Aluminum exposure is a major suspect.

You may not suffer from any of the above conditions, but that doesn't mean you haven't been poisoned by aluminum. Here is a checklist of symptoms associated with aluminum toxicity.[62] If you are experiencing two or more of them, you should try eliminating all aluminum from your kitchen immediately:

- Constipation
- Brain fog
- Anorexia
- Gastrointestinal irritation
- Hyperactivity
- Speech disorder
- Dementia
- Osteomalacia
- Headaches
- Abnormal heart rhythm
- Numbness of hands and feet
- Blurred vision
- Impaired memory

UNpacking Future Generations

Pressure from Big Chem has kept these hazardous materials on the market, even as they fall under scrutiny from an increasingly vocal group of neuroscientists,

---

[61] Nancy Mullan, et al., "Aluminum Toxicity in Mitochondrial Dysfunction and ASD."

[62] www.bodyhealth.com/sources-heavy-metals.

toxicologists, endocrinologists, biochemists, and pediatricians. As we have seen, their trailblazing studies
are turning up uncomfortable truths. One particularly
disturbing discovery is that many infants today are
born with heavy metals in their systems. Aluminum,
tin, and other toxic metals can pass to the baby from
breast milk or the placenta.[63] BPA has been shown to
gather in a particularly high concentration in the placenta. Although it is unclear how much BPA passes
from mother to child, the National Toxicology Program,
which has been studying BPA extensively since 2008,
has concluded there is "some concern" of developmental toxicity in fetuses, infants, and children.[64] A 2011
study even found that mothers with high levels of BPA
in their urine were more likely to have daughters with
hyperactivity, anxiety, and depression. These symptoms began showing up with girls as young as 3 years
old.[65]

---

[63] www.positivehealth.com/article/environmental/heavy-metal-
toxicity-an-unsuspected-illness.

[64] www.infantrisk.com/content/bisphenol-effects.

[65] Joe M. Braun, et al., "Impact of Early-Life Bisphenol A Exposure
on Behavior and Executive Function in Children," *Pediatrics* 128.5
(2011): 873–82.

In his *New York Times* editorial "Big Chem, Big Harm?," Nicholas Kristof discusses how the effects of these chemicals might be epigenetic, meaning that chemical exposure to an adult may effect their future offspring. "It's scary," said Jennifer T. Wolstenholme of the University of Virginia, who has found that the descendants of mice exposed to low doses of BPA (comparable to amounts of human consumption) exhibited behavior that parallels autism and ADHD. "These results at low doses add profoundly to concerns about endocrine disruptors," said John Peterson Myers, chief scientist at Environmental Health Sciences. "It's going to be harder than just eliminating exposure to one generation." Kristof hopes these new studies vault the issue onto the national stage. "Threats to us need to be addressed," he pleads, "even if they come not from Iranian nuclear weapons, but from things as banal as canned soup and A.T.M. receipts."[66]

The UNpacked Diet™ may well be the only diet that will actually improve your own health *and* that of future generations. If we can move toward an UNpacked society, we can change the course of our growing obesity epidemic, reverse increasing rates of chronic illness, and save our children from deadly mistakes they never chose to make.

UNpack your pounds, UNpack your potential, UNpack your food!

The UNpacked Diet™ has proven results to make you look and feel better than you have in years. By avoiding the toxins, obesogens, and carcinogens commonly found in food packaging, you will quickly detoxify your body.

---

[66] www.nytimes.com/2012/08/26/opinion/sunday/kristof-big-chem-big-harm.html?_r=0.

NO STICK? NO PROBLEM! Teflon, a common nonstick coating for pans was once thought to be a cancer-causing agent. Numerous studies have debunked this myth. In fact, due to Teflon's nonstick nature, food actually has less contact with the cooking surface, making it one of the safest culinary materials around.

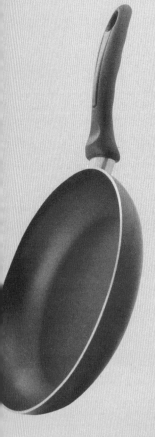

Most diets promise you the freedom to eat "whatever you want" but follow that promise with a list of restricted foods. The UNpacked Diet™ has no such list. It is compatible with any culinary tradition and allows all categories of food. You will never have to sit out on that chocolate cake or avoid the bread basket again! You will never feel embarrassed or left out because of your elimination diet. You will find that eating supposedly unhealthy foods you avoided for years will make you feel great, as long as they are free from the contamination of packaging.

It's that simple.

Eat what you want, as much as you want, whenever you want, as long as you adhere to the following rules:

- Avoid food that has been stored in sealed plastic or plastic wrap. Choose breathable plastic containers (fruit clamshells/produce bags) over tighter wraps, and use cloth mesh bags to gather loose produce.

- Beware of boxed foods with hidden plastic bags (cereal, cracker and cookie boxes are common offenders). Check paper bags for plastic linings. You can never be too careful!

- Store leftovers in glass or ceramic containers. Use UNpacked™ nonporous liners to reduce contamination.

- Never reheat food in plastic.

- Avoid canned or tinned foods. Remember: "BPA-free" containers have plastic lining and contain toxic metals.

- Never drink hot liquids from plastic or Styrofoam cups/bowls.

- Cook smart: Don't taint chemical-free foods with shavings from plastic cutting boards or overheated spatulas. Use wood or bamboo boards and wood or stainless steel utensils.

- Avoid cereals, pasta, rice, etc. packaged in recycled cardboard boxes, which have been proven to contain carcinogenic mineral oils.

- Use cloth or unbleached paper tea bags. Use unbleached coffee filters, and only UNpacked™–approved coffeemakers.

- Never store leftover food in direct contact with aluminum foil or in aluminum containers/ pans.

- Don't cook/bake with aluminum pans or bake using aluminum foil. Never put foil on the grill.

- Keep vitamins/supplements safe using UNpacked™ nonporous liners.

(UNpacked™ nonporous liners, a list of UNpacked™–approved coffeemakers, and the UNpacked™ Cookbook *are all available at unpackeddiet.com.)*

I've experienced the extraordinary benefits of this diet myself. No more acne, no more dry skin, no more brain fog. Now that I understand the science, I'm no longer scared of getting cancer, Alzheimer's, or any of the diseases that modern medicine wants to treat with medication. You don't have to be scared either. And my

man boobs—yes, I admit I had them!—went away completely, thanks to getting all that synthetic estrogen out
of my system.

But don't take my word for it. Here are actual testimonials from people who have gone UNpacked:

*"I pre-ordered this book, and finally went unpacked one week
before the book was released. And what a difference. My blood
pressure had been averaging 140/88 (taking two blood pressure medications). Now, after only two weeks of unpacked
eating, I've averaged 124/68 for the past four days. I've reduced one of my medications to keep my blood pressure from
dropping too low after it fell to 108/58. It's crazy! And I'm not
starving myself. I'm getting plenty to eat."*

*"My husband and I immediately changed to the unpacked way
of eating and subsequently in just a matter of a few weeks I
have lost 16 lbs. I am not fat AT ALL. But my weight had crept
up over the last couple of years and I couldn't seem to get it
back down to normal for me. I feel GREAT! My parents are also
on this way of eating. They are in their 70s, very active, health
conscious, and very open minded."*

"I started to eat unpacked, and my energy was not only soaring, but my depression lifted, my skin became smoother and softer, and I dropped down to a size 4 without even trying to lose weight! (I've never been less than a size 10 in my life!) Anyways, I effortlessly maintained that level of vitality and a size 4 until I started to eat packaged rice flour, oats, meats and candy. I quickly gained 15lbs and fell into depression once again, leading me to realize that once on an unpacked diet, it must become a way of life."

"At 49 years old and 245 lbs I knew I needed to do something to change my health for the better. This program changed everything for me, my health, my weight, my pain . . . I felt 30 years younger, no pain at all and I have Fibromyalgia. 40 days and I ended up 35 lbs lighter, slept like a baby, no more pain. . . I could hardly walk I was in so much pain. If you truly want to do something great for yourself/health this is truly is. . . . Unpacking saved my life!!!!!!!!!!!!!!!"

"I was very overweight and couldn't seem to lose it. I felt bloated and 'puffy' as well as having no energy. Due to all this I was lacking in confidence and had a poor self-image. I found the Unpacked Diet and I committed to following it.

"In 10 days I lost 22 pounds (10 kg). I was feeling so good I continued on following the diet plan and lost 55 pounds (25 kg) in 3 months and regained all my energy and self-esteem. My Mum is so impressed she is now following the diet."

"This is unbelievable. The hardest part was releasing all the 'diet rules' that I've picked up over the years and just learn to listen to the Unpacked Diet. The first day I did what Levino-vitz suggested, I lost 4 lbs - no joke! . . . I'd recommend this to anyone who is tired of yo-yo dieting. You never have to restrict yourself again. This is awesome!"

So Try UNpacking for Just 30 Days— What Do You Have to Lose Besides Your Weight?

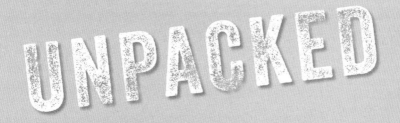

The UNpacked Diet™

UNpack your pounds. UNpack your potential. UNpack your food.

Finally: a scientifically proven revolution in healthy eating!

- Learn why what you eat isn't the problem.

- Learn why nutritionists and scientists always disagree about which foods are bad and which foods are good.

- Stop listening to the hype and start living the truth.

- Embrace the UNpacked Diet™ . . . and say goodbye to fad diets forever!

> This intro section is adapted from Dr. Mark Hyman's *10-Day Detox*. The list of ailments is the same. It uses nine days instead of ten because nine is a lucky Chinese number.

UNpacked 9-Day Detox

Here's my promise: With JUST 9 days on the UNpacked Diet, you'll be jump-started on the path to health. Some people, including doctors, don't think you can radically transform your health in a few days, but I do. Why? Because I've seen it happen with my own eyes. Just follow my proven program, and in 9 days not only can you lose up to 9 pounds, but you can also prevent or reverse chronic health problems including diabetes, asthma, joint pain, digestive problems, auto-immune disease, headaches, brain fog, allergies, acne, eczema, and even sexual dysfunction.

Step One: Be Honest With Yourself

> Makes the reader incredibly insecure and vulnerable.

Weigh yourself. Measure your waistline. Then think back to the last time you felt completely rested and fully energized. Now, ask yourself: Is this the real you, or is someone different—leaner, smarter, happier, better—hidden inside, trying to escape? Are you ready to help?

Step Two: Read the UNpacked Diet

Find out what's keeping you from becoming your true self. You'll be shocked, you'll be angry, and you'll be empowered to make the changes that will start you on the road to health. Best of all—you'll be able to eat every single food you love: carbs, fats, salt, sugar, wheat, meat, dairy. Unlike other diets, when you UNpack, you really don't have to give up anything.

Step Three: 9-Day Detox

For just nine days, UNpack your diet. Then go back to step one. Weigh yourself. Measure your waistline. Then think back to the last time you felt completely rested and fully energized. Now, ask yourself: Have you started UNpacking the pounds, like so many other people have? Have you started UNpacking your potential?

Of course you have! So make the UNpacked Diet a lifestyle, not just a diet!

Why Us, Why Now?

Think back to the traditional meals your great-grandmother and grandmother prepared: huge bowls of mashed potatoes, giant beef roasts, pale bread rolls slathered in butter, fresh-baked pies with flaky lard crusts. Your parents probably have fond memories of chasing after the ice cream truck every day of summer. And we have beautiful vintage Coca-Cola ads to remind us of a time when kids guiltlessly drank a bottle of Coke whenever the days were hot.

How did they get away with eating like that, when today the same types of foods are said to cause chronic disease?

Conventional wisdom tells us that unhealthy eating habits cause the obesity, hypertension, heart disease, stroke, and diabetes that plague our modern world. New research shows that diet can also cause psychological conditions like ADHD, Alzheimer's, schizophrenia, and autism.

But which foods are the problem? Scientists and diet gurus "whiplash" us back and forth on the culprits—from salt to sugar to fat to gluten. Do you trust the Paleolithic crowd? That means red meat is fine and whole grains are dangerous. Do you trust our government? Then whole grains are a must, and red meat will give you cancer and heart disease. Mainstream nutritionists will tell you it's all about energy balance—just eat fewer calories than you burn. But if you're among those who have tried diet and exercise, you *know* there's more to the story.

Immediately invokes the myth of paradise past.

They didn't, if the implication is that life was safer back then. The age-adjusted risk of dying *dropped* 60 percent between 1935 and 2010.

Establishes the UNpacked Diet as antiestablishment, appealing to people who are frustrated with "mainstream medicine."

Refers vaguely to "new research" and fails to disclose disagreement in the scientific community about whether and how diet is connected to these problems.

Looking to traditional cultures for our optimal diet raises even more questions. We know that African Masai tribes stay disease-free on a diet of raw milk and meat.[1] Yet we attribute the great health of the ancient Chinese to their nearly vegetarian diet.[2] The Yanomamo Indians of Brazil thrive on a salt-free diet, whereas the Japanese (one of the healthiest modern cultures with virtually no heart disease) eat the highest-sodium diet in the world.[3,4]

Could it be that conventional wisdom is only *partially* right?

There is something wrong with our diet. Of course there is! Look at the skyrocketing rates of obesity, chronic disease, cancer, and mental illness.

But here's the shocking truth: the *type* of food we eat isn't the problem.

The *only* thing everyone agrees on is that sick, obese America eats too much processed and packaged food. According to a *New York Times* report, Americans eat 31 percent more packaged food than fresh food. We eat more packaged food than almost any other country. But don't jump to conclusions about what's in those packages. Nearly 40 percent of packaged-food consumption in America comes from dairy, especially heart-healthy yogurt and skim milk. Only 6 percent of our packaged-food consumption comes from those

> Reinforces the myth of paradise past and "noble savages" using unsubstantiated references to healthy traditional cultures. There is no consensus about the extent to which diet plays a role in the health of any of these cultures. Not only that, most accounts of healthy traditional cultures are outdated or anecdotal.

> Uses cherry-picked data. Excludes the information that snack and candy consumption in America is twice that of almost all other countries. Also fails to mention that overall total food consumption is highest per capita in America.

---

[1] Friedrich-Schiller-Universität Jena, "Nomadic People's Good Health Baffles Scientists," ScienceDaily, May 18, 2010.

[2] Keith Akers, *A Vegetarian Sourcebook: The Nutrition, Ecology, and Ethics of a Vegetarian Diet*, (Vegetarian Press, 1983).

[3] William J. Oliver, Edwin L. Cohen, and James V. Neel, "Blood Pressure, Sodium Intake, and Sodium Related Hormones in the Yanomamo Indians, a 'No-Salt' Culture," *Circulation* 52.1 (1975): 146–51.

[4] Taichi Shimazu, et al., "Dietary Patterns and Cardiovascular Disease Mortality in Japan: A Prospective Cohort Study," *International Journal of Epidemiology* 36.3 (2007): 600–609.

snacks and candy we associate with weight gain and disease.[5]

In fact, as food manufacturers and fast-food chains produce "healthier" options, including low-fat meals, cultured dairy, whole grain breads, and preprepared salads, our health continues to decline. It seems like the harder we try and the more we know, the worse things get.

> Simplified alarmism about general health is rarely accurate. Our life spans are longer than ever, and there is considerable scientific debate about supposed increases in conditions like ADHD, autism, and cancer.

So let's ask again: What has *really* changed since the healthier generations of our past? What do they and the Yanomamo and the Masai all have in common?

When I think of my 95-year-old grandmother, I always think of a glass jar. In fact, her kitchen was filled with them. At the end of the summer, she would stuff jars with fruits and vegetables to preserve and eat all year long.

> Anecdotes about longevity are powerful but do not constitute decisive evidence of anything.

Today, glass is infrequently used to store food, and for one simple reason: Big Food wants to keep things cheap. Gone is Grandmother's pantry. Kitchens are now filled with plastics, metals, and heavily bleached and processed papers. Many people have never even seen a traditional burlap sack. Instead, our rice and grains are sealed into plastic bags. Milk, which once came delivered fresh in glass jugs, sits for days in plastic containers or plastic-lined cartons. Our grandparents brought fresh produce home in crates and cartons. We get our fruits and veggies precut, conveniently shrink-wrapped in plastic and Styrofoam.

> Evokes a narrative of good and evil in which anything associated with industry must be bad.

> Appeals to fear of modernity.

Our Paleolithic ancestors ate a wide variety of diets depending on where they lived.[6] But none of them

---

[5] www.nytimes.com/imagepates/2010/04/04/business/04metrics_g.html.

[6] Marlene Zuk, *Paleofantasy: What Evolution Really Tells Us about Sex, Diet, and How We Live* (New York: W. W. Norton & Company, 2013).

> Contrasts modernity with an idealized vision of Nature with a capital *N*.

shopped at grocery stores. They found their food in Nature, wrapped in Nature's packaging of peels and husks. Food today is a different story. Wherever it is found, from gas station mini-marts to giant Walmarts, it almost always comes packaged. And even when it doesn't, we place it in plastic bags ourselves before taking it home to feed our families.

If we are willing to ignore old ways of thinking about food, the answer to our dietary problems is obvious. The whiplash goes away when we stop trying to figure which *type* of food is the dietary villain, or which new fad diet will help us lose weight and get rid of chronic disease. Science can't tell us which diet is right because there *isn't* a right diet!

Here's what science can tell us, and it's what all those whiplashing diet gurus and nutritionists don't want you know, because they'd be out of a job. The most common supermarket and fast-food materials—plastic, aluminum, tin, even recycled paper—contain dangerous chemicals and heavy metals that fatten us up and destroy our health.

> Identifies a satisfyingly simple scapegoat to blame for all our health problems.

The real villain is in the packaging.

Plastics Are Not Fantastic

> Uses pseudo-scientific jargon. Nanoplastic is a real term, but it does not mean "small plastic particles." It sure sounds scary, though.
>
> Big Chem and Big Food = Supervillains!

The dangers of plastics are no surprise to scientists, who have been studying their negative health effects for decades. Researchers and health officials have voiced concerns about "nanoplastics" (small plastic particles) that get into our food by "leaching" or "migration." Although Big Chem and Big Food have done their best to suppress this information, numerous studies prove the health risks are enormous.

Unlike low carb vs. low fat, there is no debate about the dangers of these modern food storage materials.

> False.

You may have heard about the most notorious of these plastics, BPA. Polycarbonate plastics (containing BPA) are extremely common in US food packaging. In 2004, the CDC found traces of BPA in nearly all the urine samples it collected (93 percent of adults), and scientists predict that today the number would be over 99 percent.[7] The source of this BPA is primarily our diets.[8]

> Seems alarming, but there are traces of many things in our bodies that are dangerous at higher doses. The dose makes the poison.

The dangers of this poisonous endocrine disrupter are almost too numerous to list. BPA mimics estrogen and has been shown to grow breast cancer cells.[9] Exposure to BPA early in life leads to precancerous changes in the prostate and mammary glands, altered brain development, lower sperm counts, chromosomal abnormalities in eggs, obesity, and insulin resistance.[10] Prenatal exposure to BPA correlates with breast cancer later in life, a fact so alarming that the Breast Cancer Fund urges people to avoid *all BPA plastics*.[11] They also recommend eliminating canned food, since BPA is commonly used in can lining.[12]

> The terrifying associations made in this paragraph are based on a few in-vitro and animal studies. Establishing facts about what causes cancer in humans requires many human studies and epidemiological studies.
>
> Based on a single study, conducted on primates, with very tentative conclusions.
>
> Organizations don't always make recommendations based on sound science. The Breast Cancer Fund is basing their recommendations on the kind of studies mentioned above.

---

[7] Antonia M. Calafat, et al., "Exposure of the US population to Bisphenol A and 4-Tertiary-Octylphenol: 2003–2004," *Environmental Health Perspectives* (2008): 39–44.

[8] L Trasande, TM Attina, and J Blustein, "Association between Urinary Bisphenol A Concentration and Obesity Prevalence in Children and Adolescents," *JAMA* 308 (2012): 1113–21.

[9] Endocrine Society, "BPA Stimulates Growth of an Advanced Subtype of Human Breast Cancer Cells Called Inflammatory Breast Cancer," ScienceDaily, June 23, 2014.

[10] www.medicalnewstoday.com/articles/243626.php.

[11] Endocrine Society, "BPA Exposure in Utero May Increase Predisposition to Breast Cancer," ScienceDaily, October 3, 2011.

[12] www.breastcancerfund.org/reduce-your-risk/tips/eat-live-better.

> Just because a study isn't funded by industry doesn't mean it is reliable or free of bias.
>
> If the highest levels of BPA are still safe, then this doesn't matter. The "highest" levels identified in the study still fall well below the FDA's guidelines and even the more conservative EPA limits.

Just think about the implications for so-called healthy eaters. An independent, nonindustry Breast Cancer Fund study looked at more than 300 products and found BPA levels were highest in some of the "healthiest" low-calorie foods such as canned vegetables, soup, and lite coconut milk.[13] That puts those who think they are making smart food choices at the highest risk.

Thankfully, BPA buildup may be reversible. In 2011, the Breast Cancer Fund, in conjunction with the Silent Spring Institute, put a BPA detox diet to the test. Their study, published in *Environmental Health Perspectives* (a prestigious journal overseen by the National Institute of Health), tested families who adopted a diet that eliminated all packaged foods. By the end of the study, BPA levels had dropped by an astonishing 60 percent![14]

> Great example of nonindustry bias. Here are some quotes from the Silent Spring website, illustrating their distrust of scientific methodology and impatience with the scientific process:
>
> *"[The Silent Spring Institute] decided to create a laboratory of their own. . . . Their background was social activism, not science—and that gave them an advantage."*
>
> *"We didn't want science as usual. We didn't want to fund scientists that would go away and then come back with a report ten years later."*
>
> Published studies in prestigious journals aren't always reliable. See the following comment:
>
> Five families participated in the study. The diet lasted for three days.

---

[13] Breast Cancer Fund (2010), What Labels Don't Tell Us: Getting BPA out of Our Food and Our Bodies, www.breastcancerfund.org/assets/pdfs/publications/what-labels-dont-tell-us-1.pdf.

[14] Ruthann A. Rudel, et al., "Food Packaging and Bisphenol A and Bis (2-Ethyhexyl) Phthalate Exposure: Findings from a Dietary Intervention," *Environmental Health Perspectives* 119.7 (2011): 914–20.

WOULD YOU LIKE YOUR RECEIPT? Cash register receipts are coated with BPA, which absorbs into the skin. If you are highly BPA-sensitive, consider shopping with gloves or declining the receipt.

Considered toxic in Canada and outlawed across the European Union, it's amazing that BPA is still used at all. Although the FDA has finally banned BPA from baby bottles, Big Food and Big Chem continue to fight against further regulation. Instead, they encourage us to focus on "healthy foods," cranking out low-cal, low-fat product lines that depend on the cheap packaging that's at the heart of our nation's health problems.

Frighteningly, BPA is just the tip of the iceberg. Another 2011 study from *Environmental Health Perspectives* tested 500 chemical containers and found that nearly all of them, even those previously considered safe, release estrogen-mimicking chemicals. BPA-free products, including baby bottles, actually release synthetic estrogens that are *more potent than BPA!*[15] Stuart Yaniger, one of the lead authors of the study, put it bluntly: "Baby bottles, plastic bags, plastic wrap, clamshell food containers, stand-up pouches: Just about anything you can think of that's made of plastic that food or beverages are wrapped up in, we found this activity. It was shocking to us."[16]

As we saw with MSG and salt, regulatory action, especially when it comes to infant safety, often jumps the gun and creates the illusion of a scientific consensus. In a 2012 press release, the FDA stated that the reason for their BPA ban was "abandonment," which means companies had stopped the practice of using BPA in infant bottles. The release included the explicit statement that "safety information is not relevant to abandonment."

It's one thing to say containers release chemicals. It's quite another to prove a connection between those chemicals and health problems.

[15] *Environmental Health Perspectives* 119 (2011): 989–96. dx.doi.org/10.1289/ehp.1003220. [online March 2, 2011]

[16] www.chriskresser.com/how-plastic-food-containers-could-be-making-you-fat-infertile-and-sick.

Yaniger's warning about plastic wrap is particularly important. Plastic wraps are known to contain an extremely dangerous endocrine disrupter called DEHA (diethyl hexyl adipate). Panicked industry groups continue to deny its toxicity, but unbiased researchers keep linking DEHA to liver tumors, asthma, and cancer.[17] Consumers Union research confirmed that food wrapped in plastic, like deli cheeses, had DEHA levels exceeding levels considered safe in Europe.[18] You wouldn't wrap your food in a poison-soaked cloth, but that's exactly what you're doing when you wrap your food in plastic contaminated with DEHA.

> Stuart Yaniger works for PlastiPure, a company with a product line of plastics whose mission is to ensure "that estrogenic chemicals will not leach into foods, drinks, and other materials." That doesn't mean his study is wrong—but it does mean we should extend the same skepticism to him that we would to an industry-funded study asserting the safety of plastics.
>
> Supplying the full scientific name means nothing, but it helps to establish expertise and invoke fear of modernity.
>
> Remember, just because industry denies something doesn't mean the opposite is true.
>
> In their report, the Consumers Union also emphasized that the risks were small.
>
> "Safe in Europe . . ." True, but who cares? Legal safety levels for chemicals can differ drastically between countries and public health organizations, and routinely have no basis in sound science.

[17] www.center4research.org/healthy-living-prevention/products-with-health-risks/plastic-wrap-and-plastic-food-containers-are-they-safe.

[18] www.consumersunion.org/news/report-to-the-fda-regarding-plastic-packaging.

As use of plastic increases, so do rates of mental disorders like ADHD and autism.[19] While the two seem intuitively unrelated, scientists see a connection. Irva Hertz-Picciotto, chief of the Division of Environmental and Occupational health at UC Davis, believes that because plastic packaging interferes with the body's natural hormonal system, it could "play a role in autism or other neurodevelopmental disorders." Other doctors suspect plastic packaging may disrupt thyroid hormone, which is critical for brain development. Thyroid dysfunction is particularly common in children with autism.[20]

> This is highly controversial. Many experts have suggested that rates of autism are not, in fact, rising, and better detection and expanded criteria account for the perceived "epidemic."
>
> It could play a role . . . or it could not.
>
> It may . . . or it may not.

And those migraines? They aren't just in your head. According to the Mayo Clinic, plastics may be responsible for your migraine. The hormones estrogen and progesterone play key roles in regulating menstruation and pregnancy, which affect headache-causing chemicals in the brain.[21] Steady estrogen levels improve headaches, but altered levels make them worse. A University of Kansas study found that hormone-disrupting plastics caused migraine symptoms, including light and sound sensitivity.[22] Chemicals in plastic food packaging have also been linked to heart disease,[23] adult

> . . . in rats.

> Lots of citations doesn't mean good science. Every "link" in this sentence is based on a single study, sometimes with very tenuous conclusions.

---

[19] www.articles.mercola.com/sites/articles/archive/2014/04/02/environmental-toxin-exposure.aspx.

[20] www.thechart.blogs.cnn.com/2011/06/07/scientists-warn-of-chemical-autism-link.

[21] www.mayoclinic.org/diseases-conditions/chronic-daily-headaches/in-depth/headaches/art-20046729.

[22] NEJ Berman, E Gregory, KE McCarson et al., "Exposure to Bisphenol A Exacerbates Migraine-Like Behaviors in a Multibehavior Model of Rat Migraine," *Toxicological Sciences* 137.2 (2014): 416–27.

[23] Naomi Lubick, "Cardiovascular Health: Exploring a Potential Link between BPA and Heart Disease," *Environmental Health Perspectives* 118.3 (2010): A116.

onset diabetes,[24] high blood pressure,[25] early puberty,[26] allergies,[27] asthma,[28] anxiety,[29] unattractiveness,[30] erectile dysfunction,[31] depression,[32] schizophrenia,[33] and Alzheimer's.[34]

So plastics make us sick—but do they also make us fat? The answer is clear. Scientists have known for over a decade that plastics cause obesity in rats, and recently found that the link extends to humans. In the 2012 Smithsonian.com article "Is the Can Worse Than the Soda?" author Joseph Stromberg cites the first

[24] Ben Harder, "Diabetes from a Plastic?: Estrogen Mimic Provokes Insulin Resistance," *Science News* 169.3 (2006): 36–37.

[25] Leonardo Trasande, et al., "Urinary Phthalates Are Associated with Higher Blood Pressure in Childhood," *Journal of Pediatrics* 163.3 (2013): 747–53.

[26] Jonathan R. Roy, Sanjoy Chakraborty, and Tandra R. Chakraborty, "Estrogen-Like Endocrine Disrupting Chemicals Affecting Puberty in Humans: A Review," *Medical Science Monitor* 15.6 (2009): 137–45.

[27] Datis Kharrazian, "The Potential Roles of Bisphenol A (BPA) Pathogenesis in Autoimmunity," *Autoimmune Diseases*, vol. 2014, Article ID 743616, 12 pages, 2014. doi:10.1155/2014/743616.

[28] Carl-Gustaf Bornehag, et al., "The Association between Asthma and Allergic Symptoms in Children and Phthalates in House Dust: A Nested Case-Control Study," *Environmental Health Perspectives* (2004): 1393–97.

[29] Bryce C. Ryan, and John G. Vandenbergh, "Developmental Exposure to Environmental Estrogens Alters Anxiety and Spatial Memory in Female Mice." *Hormones and Behavior* 50.1 (2006): 85–93.

[30] Lisa A. M. Galea, and Cindy K. Barha, "Maternal Bisphenol A (BPA) Decreases Attractiveness of Male Offspring," *Proceedings of the National Academy of Sciences* 108.28 (2011): 11305–6.

[31] De-Kun Li, et al., "Relationship between Urine Bisphenol-A Level and Declining Male Sexual Function," *Journal of Andrology* 31.5 (2010): 500–506.

[32] www.rodalenews.com/multiple-chemical-sensitivity.

[33] James S. Brown, "Effects of Bisphenol-A and Other Endocrine Disruptors Compared with Abnormalities of Schizophrenia: An Endocrine-Disruption Theory of Schizophrenia," *Schizophrenia Bulletin* 35.1 (2009): 256–78.

[34] Wei Sun, et al., "Perinatal Exposure to Di-(2-Ethylhexyl)-Phthalate Leads to Cognitive Dysfunction and Phospho-Tau Level Increase in Aged Rats," *Environmental Toxicology* (2012).

large-scale study (with a sample of around 3,000 children) to find a significant link between BPA and obesity. Stromberg notes the study "hints at the surprisingly complex root causes of obesity, once thought to simply reflect an imbalance between caloric intake and exercise."[35] A later study in the journal *Pediatrics* looked at 3,300 children ages six to eighteen and found that those with high BPA levels tended to have "excessive amounts of body fat and unusually expanded waistlines."[36] A 2013 study by Kaiser Permanente found that girls with higher levels of BPA were *five times more likely to be overweight*.[37] Several studies have linked plastics to expanded waistlines and insulin resistance. One 2013 study in *Environmental Health Perspectives* found plastic exposure put African American children especially at risk for obesity. The authors reported that every unit increase of nanoplastics in their urine meant a 21 percent higher chance the child would be overweight and 22 percent higher chance the child would be obese.[38]

It is no coincidence that when plastic use took off, we started packing on the pounds.

> Correlation is not causation.

> Stromberg also notes that "the finding is only a correlation between the amount of BPA in the body and obesity, rather than evidence that one causes the other."

> . . . *high BPA levels tended* . . .
>
> Correlation is not causation!

> False. Very likely a coincidence.

Styrofoam: A Heated Debate

Polystyrene, familiar to most of us as Styrofoam, is technically a type of plastic. It is commonly used for drinking cups, fast-food packaging, egg cartons, and takeout

[35] www.smithsonianmag.com/ist/?next=/science-nature/is-the-can-worse-than-the-soda-study-finds-correlation-between-bpa-and-obesity-40894828.

[36] Donna S. Eng, et al., "Bisphenol A and Chronic Disease Risk Factors in US Children," *Pediatrics* 132.3 (2013): e637–e645.

[37] De-Kun Li, Maohua Miao, ZhiJun Zhou, Chunhua Wu, Huijing Shi, Xiaoqin Liu, Siqi Wang, and Wei Yuan, "Urine Bisphenol-A Level in Relation to Obesity and Overweight in School-Age Children," *PLoS ONE*, 2013; 8 (6): e65399 DOI: 10.1371/journal.pone.0065399.

[38] Leonardo Trasande, et al., "Race/Ethnicity-Specific Associations of Urinary Phthalates with Childhood Body Mass in a Nationally Representative Sample," *Environmental Health Perspectives* 121.4 (2013): 501–506.

boxes. Although you find it everywhere, polystyrene foam contains styrene, which is a known carcinogen. A study of more than 12,000 male workers in a styrene polymer factory found styrene-exposed workers had an increased risk of leukemia and non-Hodgkin's lymphoma. The digestive system seems particularly susceptible to harm from styrene, as researchers also found higher rates of esophageal cancer in Caucasians and stomach cancer in blacks. Black workers exposed to styrene also had higher rates of heart disease.[39] Other observed health risks from styrene exposure include irritation of the skin, eyes, upper respiratory tract, and gastrointestinal problems.[40] That's not to mention "styrene sickness," a condition characterized by headaches, fatigue, brain fog, and depression.[41]

It is well documented that hot liquids cause Styrofoam to melt and break down. Health authorities say to never heat Styrofoam cups in the microwave, and warn against using them with warm beverages.[42] Yet Big Food continues to use polystyrene for their hot beverages and soups, and we keep drinking their products. One of the worst offenders is Dunkin' Donuts, which uses about 1 billion Styrofoam cups each year. There have been several petitions and a Facebook group dedicated to changing Dunkin' Donuts' packaging, but so far the company has resisted.[43] All along you've been wary of those trans-fat-filled doughnuts, when your Styrofoam

> Almost completely irrelevant. These factory workers were breathing in large quantities of styrene. The monotonic fallacy—if a lot is bad, a little is also bad—comes into play.

> Inhaled styrene's harm to the digestive system does not mean that ingesting small amounts of styrene is likely to be harmful.

> Which health authorities? Turns out mostly alarmist, unreliable ones. Has your doctor ever mentioned this to you?

> These movements generally focus on environmental concerns, not health concerns.

[39] Genevieve M. Matanoski, Carlos Santos-Burgoa, and Linda Schwartz, "Mortality of a Cohort of Workers in the Styrene-Butadiene Polymer Manufacturing Industry (1943–1982)," *Environmental Health Perspectives* 86 (1990): 107.

[40] www.earthresource.org/campaigns/capp/capp-styrofoam.html.

[41] www.rodalenews.com/coffee-and-styrofoam-cups.

[42] www.ewg.org/research/healthy-home-tips/tip-3-pick-plastics-carefully.

[43] www.facebook.com/pages/Encouraging-Dunkin-Donuts-to-stop-using-1-Billion-styrofoam-cups-a-year/199731989943.

KNOW YOUR PAPER. A paper cup can be a great safe alternative when you're on the go and forget your mug. But not all paper is created equal. Recycled paper in cereal boxes has been shown to cause cancer. Chlorine-bleached paper tea bags contain dioxin, a known carcinogen that can seep into your hot liquid.

coffee cup is the real killer. Can you believe it? Your Dunkin' coffee is worse than your Dunkin' Donut. Remember: *America dies on Dunkin'*!

But it turns out coffee is just a drop in the (plastic) bucket. Our greatest source of chemical disrupters comes from bottled water. Americans consume more than 9 billion gallons of bottled water a year, and rates are rising fast.[44] Although they don't look like Styrofoam, water bottles are made from polystyrene plastic. A 2006 study found high levels of styrene in brand-new bottled water samples. The levels increased over time as the bottled water sat on the shelf. When the bottles were heated, the levels were even higher, but even in fresh, cold water, the results were alarming![45] A later study published in the journal *Environmental Science and Pollution Research* confirmed that there were endocrine-disrupting chemicals in all the bottled water samples tested.[46]

> The big number sounds excessive, but only without comparison data from other countries. Like our salt consumption, American bottled water consumption is lower than that of many other countries, including Mexico, Thailand, Italy, Belgium, Germany, the United Arab Emirates, and France.

> High levels are not alarming if they have no health implications.

> They never confirmed that the levels were toxic. *The dose makes the poison.*

---

[44] "Smaller categories still saw growth as the U.S. liquid refreshment beverage market shrunk by 2.0 percent in 2008, Beverage Marketing Corporation reports," press release, Beverage Marketing Corporation, March 30, 2009.

[45] Maqbool Ahmad and Ahmad S. Bajahlan, "Leaching of Styrene and Other Aromatic Compounds in Drinking Water from PS Bottles," *Journal of Environmental Sciences* 19.4 (2007): 421–26.

[46] Martin Wagner and Jörg Oehlmann, "Endocrine Disruptors in Bottled Mineral Water: Total Estrogenic Burden and Migration from Plastic Bottles," *Environmental Science and Pollution Research* 16.3 (2009): 278–86.

The following chart tracks bottled water consumption, and the curve almost exactly matches the growth of our obesity epidemic! Dietitians emphasize that drinking plenty of water is key to weight loss. Yet it's clear that drinking from bottles causes more than increased water weight.

As many of us strive to be healthy and hydrate, we find ourselves getting fatter and sicker. We drink our coffee black, without sugar or creamer, but that doesn't seem to help. We eat less at dinner and take the rest home in a takeout container, hoping to reduce our waistlines by reducing the size of our meals. But the sad truth is that all this focus on food is distracting us from the scientifically proven cause of our problems.

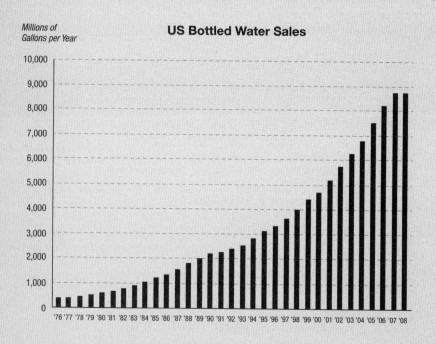

Data from the US Department of Agriculture, Economic Research Service, and the Beverage Marketing Corporation.

Correlation does not equal causation. The website Tylervigen
.com allows you to generate custom charts like these. Example:
Per capita consumption of cheese from 2000–09 correlates
almost exactly with "number of people who died by becoming
tangled in their bedsheets."

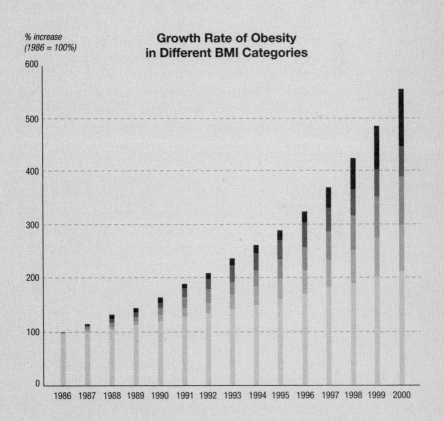

**Growth Rate of Obesity
in Different BMI Categories**

% increase
(1986 = 100%)

Legend:
- BMI ≥ 50
- BMI ≥ 45
- BMI ≥ 40
- BMI ≥ 35
- BMI ≥ 30

Source: R. Sturm, "Increases in clinically severe obesity in the
United States,1986–2000," *Arch. Intern. Med.* 163 (2003): 2146–49.

Aluminum Foiled

You might think that aluminum foil is a safe alternative for wrapping up home-cooked leftovers, but that's not true. One of the most dangerous metals lurking in our homes is aluminum.

Aluminum packaging wasn't in use until the twentieth century and is becoming increasingly popular. Global aluminum production today exceeds all metals except iron.[47] Although everyone has some amount of aluminum in the body, it provides no benefit or function. Aluminum accumulation, however, can be toxic. Aluminum has long been understood as a contributor to Alzheimer's disease, and numerous studies have confirmed the connection.[48] Scientists have found aluminum at the core of brain plaques associated with Alzheimer's.[49] But the dangers go beyond that well-known association. Aluminum exposure has been linked to everything from breast cancer to osteoporosis.[50,51] In fact, aluminum has been found to negatively inhibit more than 200 biological functions.[52]

Just as plastic leaches chemicals, research has shown that hazardous metals migrate into food when it is in contact with aluminum. So much aluminum gets into our food that the country of Oman banned cooking with it in 2010 and restricts hot food contact to the shiny side only.[53] A 1996 Italian study first brought

> Neither were air conditioners nor many vaccines. Fear of modernity, again.

> It has also "long been" controversial. There is no consensus on the connection between aluminum and Alzheimer's.

> *The dose makes the poison. The dose makes the poison. The dose makes the poison.*

[47] www.commodities-now.com/news/metals-and-mining/612-world-metal-production-surges.html.

[48] www.whfoods.com/genpage.php?tname=newtip&dbid=8.

[49] www.doctoroz.com/article/your-brain-protection-plan.

[50] P. D. Darbre, "Underarm Cosmetics Are a Cause of Breast Cancer," *European Journal of Cancer Prevention* 10.5 (2001): 389–94.

[51] Bengt Mjöberg, et al., "Aluminum, Alzheimer's Disease and Bone Fragility." *Acta Orthopaedica* 68.6 (1997): 511–14.

[52] Masahiro Kawahara and Midori Kato-Negishi, "Link between Aluminum and the Pathogenesis of Alzheimer's Disease: The Integration of the Aluminum and Amyloid Cascade Hypotheses," *International Journal of Alzheimer's Disease* (2011).

[53] www.thenational.ae/news/uae-news/aluminium-foil-linked-to-osteoporosis-and-alzheimers.

TIN CANS: THE SAFER ALTERNATIVE? Tin and aluminum are both popular canning materials. Tin exposure can cause skin and eye irritation, as well as neurological problems. And once a tin can is opened and the lining exposed to oxygen, corrosion occurs rapidly, releasing even more tin into your food.

alarm when it found 2–6 milligrams of aluminum transferred into food from foil, cookware, and utensils.[54] Follow-up studies have found even higher levels. A 2011 study in the *International Journal of Electrochemical Science* found that levels of aluminum were in toxic amounts well above the WHO safe limits in foods after they were cooked, reheated, or even simply cooled in aluminum foil. This effect was amplified by acidity—a point we will return to in a moment.[55]

Recently, scientists have directed their attention to the link between aluminum and obesity. Along with BPA in soda can liners, aluminum also helps pack on the pounds. High levels of aluminum in the body have been linked to iron deficiency, disproportionately common in those with obesity.[56] Biochemists in a 2007 report found that aluminum-induced mitochondrial dysfunction leads to obesity.[57]

Gigantic logical leaps that no reputable scientist would ever endorse.

A single in-vitro study proves nothing.

[54] L. Gramiccioni, et al., "Aluminium Levels in Italian Diets and in Selected Foods from Aluminium Utensils." *Food Additives & Contaminants* 13.7 (1996): 767–74.

[55] F. S. Mohammad, E. A. H. Al Zubaidy, and G. Bassion, "Effect of Aluminum Leaching Process of Cooking Wares on Food," *International Journal of Electrochemical Science* 6.1 (2011): 222–230.

[56] Sungwon Han, et al., "How Aluminum, an Intracellular ROS Generator Promotes Hepatic and Neurological Diseases: The Metabolic Tale," *Cell Biology and Toxicology* 29.2 (2013): 75–84.

[57] Ryan Mailloux, Joseph Lemire, and Vasu Appanna, "Aluminum-Induced Mitochondrial Dysfunction Leads to Lipid Accumulation in Human Hepatocytes: A Link to Obesity," *Cellular Physiology and Biochemistry* 20.5 (2008): 627–38.

False. Diet sodas have not been found to contribute to weight gain, except insofar as those who drink them might also consume more calories.

All this might help explain why diet sodas have been found to contribute to weight gain, a mystery that no nutrition experts can solve.[58] Remember how acidity amplifies the aluminum-leaching effect? A highly acidic zero-calorie beverage will still leach aluminum at a high rate. If you want to lose weight, you might be better off drinking a milk shake from a glass than a can of diet soda.

Then again, that's totally insane.

Ah, Russell Blaylock. Remember him from MSG? And government conspiracy chemical trails?

Not only is this a simple correlation, but it also correlates autism with injected aluminum, not aluminum from soda cans.

Frighteningly, research has also connected aluminum to learning disabilities and autism. As early as 2009, renowned neurosurgeon Russell Blaylock was examining how aluminum creates changes in the brain.[59] In a 2012 review titled "Empirical Data Confirm Autism Symptoms Related to Aluminum and Acetaminophen Exposure," the authors note that mentions of autism "increased steadily at the end of the last century, during a period when mercury was being phased out, while aluminum adjuvant burden was being increased." In the report, they link aluminum-containing vaccines to a significant rise in "cellulitis, seizure, depression, fatigue, pain and death."[60] In an article titled "Aluminum Toxicity in Mitochondrial Dysfunction and ASD," authors Nancy Mullan, MD, and Amy Yasko, PhD, AMD, FAAIM note the "intense interest and discussion surrounding the high incidence of mitochondrial disease

Don't let degrees distract you from focusing on the argument and the science. Amy Yasko is a controversial figure who endorses completely unfounded techniques for "curing autism."

[58] Susan E. Swithers, "Artificial Sweeteners Produce the Counterintuitive Effect of Inducing Metabolic Derangements," *Trends in Endocrinology & Metabolism* 24.9 (2013): 431–41.

[59] Russell L. Blaylock, "A Possible Central Mechanism in Autism Spectrum Disorders, Part 3: The Role of Excitotoxin Food Additives and the Synergistic Effects of Other Environmental Toxins," *Alternative Therapies in Health and Medicine* 15.2 (2008): 56–60.

[60] Stephanie Seneff, Robert M. Davidson, and Jingjing Liu, "Empirical Data Confirm Autism Symptoms Related to Aluminum and Acetaminophen Exposure," *Entropy* 14.11 (2012): 2227–53.

and/or dysfunction in children with autism spectrum disorders." As there is no genetic cause of this dysfunction, attention is "turning away from genetics toward the environment."[61] Aluminum exposure is a major suspect.

These two sentences don't actually make sense. They just sound scary.

You may not suffer from any of the above conditions, but that doesn't mean you haven't been poisoned by aluminum. Here is a checklist of symptoms associated with aluminum toxicity.[62] If you are experiencing two or more of them, you should try eliminating all aluminum from your kitchen immediately:

This checklist comes from some random website that sells cleansing, detox, natural sleep, and weight-loss supplements.

Who hasn't experienced two or more of these symptoms? If you haven't, you're probably superhuman.

- Constipation
- Brain fog
- Anorexia
- Gastrointestinal irritation
- Hyperactivity
- Speech disorder
- Dementia
- Osteomalacia
- Headaches
- Abnormal heart rhythm
- Numbness of hands and feet
- Blurred vision
- Impaired memory

UNpacking Future Generations
Pressure from Big Chem has kept these hazardous materials on the market, even as they fall under scrutiny from an increasingly vocal group of neuroscientists,

---

[61] Nancy Mullan, et al., "Aluminum Toxicity in Mitochondrial Dysfunction and ASD."

[62] www.bodyhealth.com/sources-heavy-metals.

This claim and the next are from a naturopathic doctor's website. As his sources he cites a book called *Staying Healthy with Nutrition,* published by Celestial Arts of Berkeley, California, and another book, called *Medical Nutrition From Marz,* based on the "19th-century philosophy of Nature Cure."

A single study that examined correlations between BPA and highly subjective variables in three-year-olds, including "poor emotional control and inhibition."

toxicologists, endocrinologists, biochemists, and pediatricians. As we have seen, their trailblazing studies are turning up uncomfortable truths. One particularly disturbing discovery is that many infants today are born with heavy metals in their systems. Aluminum, tin, and other toxic metals can pass to the baby from breast milk or the placenta.[63] BPA has been shown to gather in a particularly high concentration in the placenta. Although it is unclear how much BPA passes from mother to child, the National Toxicology Program, which has been studying BPA extensively since 2008, has concluded there is "some concern" of developmental toxicity in fetuses, infants, and children.[64] A 2011 study even found that mothers with high levels of BPA in their urine were more likely to have daughters with hyperactivity, anxiety, and depression. These symptoms began showing up with girls as young as 3 years old.[65]

This doesn't mean BPA is toxic to fetuses, infants, and children at current levels of exposure. It means BPA *may* be toxic at *some* level of exposure, and further research is warranted.

[63] www.positivehealth.com/article/environmental/heavy-metal-toxicity-an-unsuspected-illness.

[64] www.infantrisk.com/content/bisphenol-effects.

[65] Joe M. Braun, et al., "Impact of Early-Life Bisphenol A Exposure on Behavior and Executive Function in Children," *Pediatrics* 128.5 (2011): 873–82.

In his *New York Times* editorial "Big Chem, Big Harm?," Nicholas Kristof discusses how the effects of these chemicals might be epigenetic, meaning that chemical exposure to an adult may effect their future offspring. "It's scary," said Jennifer T. Wolstenholme of the University of Virginia, who has found that the descendants of mice exposed to low doses of BPA (comparable to amounts of human consumption) exhibited behavior that parallels autism and ADHD. "These results at low doses add profoundly to concerns about endocrine disruptors," said John Peterson Myers, chief scientist at Environmental Health Sciences. "It's going to be harder than just eliminating exposure to one generation." Kristof hopes these new studies vault the issue onto the national stage. "Threats to us need to be addressed," he pleads, "even if they come not from Iranian nuclear weapons, but from things as banal as canned soup and A.T.M. receipts."[66]

> Given that it can be hard to define autism and ADHD in humans, you have to wonder about reliably diagnosing the same conditions in mice.

> *Oh no you didn't!* Kristof just compared BPA to nuclear weapons!

The UNpacked Diet™ may well be the only diet that will actually improve your own health *and* that of future generations. If we can move toward an UNpacked society, we can change the course of our growing obesity epidemic, reverse increasing rates of chronic illness, and save our children from deadly mistakes they never chose to make.

UNpack your pounds, UNpack your potential, UNpack your food!

The UNpacked Diet™ has proven results to make you look and feel better than you have in years. By avoiding the toxins, obesogens, and carcinogens commonly found in food packaging, you will quickly detoxify your body.

> You can pretty much say this at will about diet. No one will stop you.

> Detoxification is not actually anything at all.

---

[66] www.nytimes.com/2012/08/26/opinion/sunday/kristof-big-chem-big-harm.html?_r=0.

NO STICK? NO PROBLEM! Teflon, a common nonstick coating for pans was once thought to be a cancer-causing agent. Numerous studies have debunked this myth. In fact, due to Teflon's nonstick nature, food actually has less contact with the cooking surface, making it one of the safest culinary materials around.

Most diets promise you the freedom to eat "whatever you want" but follow that promise with a list of restricted foods. The UNpacked Diet™ has no such list. It is compatible with any culinary tradition and allows all categories of food. You will never have to sit out on that chocolate cake or avoid the bread basket again! You will never feel embarrassed or left out because of your elimination diet. You will find that eating supposedly unhealthy foods you avoided for years will make you feel great, as long as they are free from the contamination of packaging.

> Because of the placebo effect. Because you feel virtuous. Because you are in control. Because it forces you to start paying attention to what you eat, which will almost certainly result in weight loss. But NOT because anything about the UNpacked Diet is scientifically accurate.

It's that simple.

Eat what you want, as much as you want, whenever you want, as long as you adhere to the following rules:

> These rules will make it impossible to eat like a normal human being in our culture.

- Avoid food that has been stored in sealed plastic or plastic wrap. Choose breathable plastic containers (fruit clamshells/produce bags) over tighter wraps, and use cloth mesh bags to gather loose produce.

- Beware of boxed foods with hidden plastic bags (cereal, cracker and cookie boxes are common offenders). Check paper bags for plastic linings. You can never be too careful!

- Store leftovers in glass or ceramic containers. Use UNpacked™ nonporous liners to reduce contamination.

- Never reheat food in plastic.

- Avoid canned or tinned foods. Remember: "BPA-free" containers have plastic lining and contain toxic metals.

- Never drink hot liquids from plastic or Styrofoam cups/bowls.

- Cook smart: Don't taint chemical-free foods with shavings from plastic cutting boards or overheated spatulas. Use wood or bamboo boards and wood or stainless steel utensils.

- Avoid cereals, pasta, rice, etc. packaged in recycled cardboard boxes, which have been proven to contain carcinogenic mineral oils.

- Use cloth or unbleached paper tea bags. Use unbleached coffee filters, and only UNpacked™–approved coffeemakers.

- Never store leftover food in direct contact with aluminum foil or in aluminum containers/ pans.

- Don't cook/bake with aluminum pans or bake using aluminum foil. Never put foil on the grill.

- Keep vitamins/supplements safe using UNpacked™ nonporous liners.

(UNpacked™ nonporous liners, a list of UNpacked™–approved coffeemakers, and the UNpacked™ Cookbook *are all available at unpackeddiet.com.)*

Most diet books have some conflict of interest, not least of which is sales of the book itself.

I've experienced the extraordinary benefits of this diet myself. No more acne, no more dry skin, no more brain fog. Now that I understand the science, I'm no longer scared of getting cancer, Alzheimer's, or any of the diseases that modern medicine wants to treat with medication. You don't have to be scared either. And my man boobs—yes, I admit I had them!—went away completely, thanks to getting all that synthetic estrogen out of my system.

But don't take my word for it. Here are actual testimonials from people who have gone UNpacked:

> These are actual testimonials. But not for the UNpacked Diet. They are taken from various diet books and websites, all of which offer wildly conflicting advice, scientific rationales, and diet plans. The only change made is the substitution of "unpacked" for whatever diet plan was being described.

Testimonial for *Wheat Belly*, which recommends a low-carb, no-grain diet.

"I pre-ordered this book, and finally went unpacked one week before the book was released. And what a difference. My blood pressure had been averaging 140/88 (taking two blood pressure medications). Now, after only two weeks of unpacked eating, I've averaged 124/68 for the past four days. I've reduced one of my medications to keep my blood pressure from dropping too low after it fell to 108/58. It's crazy! And I'm not starving myself. I'm getting plenty to eat."

Testimonial for *Forks Over Knives*, a vegetarian diet book that recommends whole grains and vehemently objects to everything in *Grain Brain* and *Wheat Belly*.

"My husband and I immediately changed to the unpacked way of eating and subsequently in just a matter of a few weeks I have lost 16 lbs. I am not fat AT ALL. But my weight had crept up over the last couple of years and I couldn't seem to get it back down to normal for me. I feel GREAT! My parents are also on this way of eating. They are in their 70s, very active, health conscious, and very open minded."

"I started to eat unpacked, and my energy was not only soaring, but my depression lifted, my skin became smoother and softer, and I dropped down to a size 4 without even trying to lose weight! (I've never been less than a size 10 in my life!) Anyways, I effortlessly maintained that level of vitality and a size 4 until I started to eat packaged rice flour, oats, meats and candy. I quickly gained 15lbs and fell into depression once again, leading me to realize that once on an unpacked diet, it must become a way of life."

> Testimonial for *The Paleo Diet Revised*, which claims you can "lose weight and get healthy by eating the foods you were designed to eat."

"At 49 years old and 245 lbs I knew I needed to do something to change my health for the better. This program changed everything for me, my health, my weight, my pain . . . I felt 30 years younger, no pain at all and I have Fibromyalgia. 40 days and I ended up 35 lbs lighter, slept like a baby, no more pain. . . I could hardly walk I was in so much pain. If you truly want to do something great for yourself/health this is truly is. . . . Unpacking saved my life!!!!!!!!!!!!!!"

> Testimonial for *Fat, Sick, and Nearly Dead*, a book that recommends, among other things, juicing and juice fasts. Dr. Robert Lustig, the anti-sugar author of *Fat Chance*, warns that juicing is basically the worst thing you can do to a fruit or a vegetable.

"I was very overweight and couldn't seem to lose it. I felt bloated and 'puffy' as well as having no energy. Due to all this I was lacking in confidence and had a poor self-image. I found the Unpacked Diet and I committed to following it.

"In 10 days I lost 22 pounds (10 kg). I was feeling so good I continued on following the diet plan and lost 55 pounds (25 kg) in 3 months and regained all my energy and self-esteem. My Mum is so impressed she is now following the diet."

> Testimonial for *Daniel's Diet*, a book based on the biblical vegetarian diet adopted by the prophet Daniel. The motto is "restoring God's natural health."

Testimonial for a book called *The Eden Diet*. No further comment necessary.

"*This is unbelievable. The hardest part was releasing all the 'diet rules' that I've picked up over the years and just learn to listen to the Unpacked Diet. The first day I did what Levinovitz suggested, I lost 4 lbs - no joke! . . . I'd recommend this to anyone who is tired of yo-yo dieting. You never have to restrict yourself again. This is awesome!*"

So Try UNpacking for Just 30 Days— What Do You Have to Lose Besides Your Weight?

Acknowledgments

First, thank you to everyone who corresponded with me or partici-
pated in interviews: Jennifer Thomas, Brian Wansink, Stacey Rosen-
feld, Emily Abel, Amy Kubal, Nortin Hadler, Kristen Vorhees, Priyanka
Chugh, Kate Faasse, Fiona Crichton, Keith Petrie, The Bitchy Waiter,
Fabrizio Benedetti, Wendy Woloson, Hisham Ziauddeen, Shingo Ka-
jimura, Jack Bishop, Stephan Guyenet, Paul Rozin, Sharon Salomon,
Luc Tappy, David Katz, Yoni Freedhoff, Michael Lowe, Ann Yaktine,
Cheryl Anderson, James Hamblin, Lauren Moore, Richard Forshee,
Steven Shapin, Morton Satin, Massimo Pigliucci, Andrew Ward, Ron
Hoggan, and Paul Unschuld.

Special thanks to Peter Gibson, Philip Zeitler, and Hillel Cohen for
going above and beyond in helping me understand just how much we
don't know.

Extra-special thanks to Jay Olshansky for letting me steal "Eating
in the Fourth Dimension" (nice one, Jay!).

This book wouldn't exist if Laura Helmuth at Slate hadn't taken a
chance on me back in 2013. Nor would it exist without the faith and

hard work of the team at Regan Arts, Judith Regan's vision, and Lynne Ciccaglione's calm helpfulness. To my editor Michael Szczerban—what can I say? Every writer should be so lucky.

Megan Cather read an early, terrible version and still said nice things. Larry Haber walked me through how a doctor reads a scientific study. Running Bird was patient. Countless other friends, family members, and colleagues sent me information, talked with me, and managed to be patient and encouraging. My parents did all of the above throughout my entire life.

Finally, to my wife, who has been unfailingly supportive every step of the way: I don't know how to thank you enough.

Notes

INTRODUCTION

1. **More than 100 million Americans want to avoid gluten**: NPD Group, "Percentage of U.S. Adults Trying to Cut Down or Avoid Gluten in Their Diets Reaches New High in 2013," March 6, 2013, https://www.npd.com/wps/portal/npd/us/news/press-releases/percentage-of-us-adults-trying-to-cut-down-or-avoid-gluten-in-their-diets-reaches-new-high-in-2013-reports-npd.

1. **has asked if modern "super-gluten" is a dietary demon**: Dr. Hyman is all over the place on gluten. At times he indicates that it's only bad for 20 million Americans. At other times, he implies it is killing us all. See "Dr. Hyman Discusses Gluten on the Dr. Oz Show," "Gluten: What You Don't Know Might Kill You," and "Three Hidden Ways Wheat Makes You Fat," all on drhyman.com.

1. **BREAD IS MY CRACK!**: William Davis, *Wheat Belly: Lose the Wheat, Lose the Weight, and Find Your Path Back to Health* (Emmaus, PA: Rodale, 2011), 44.

1. **it's a sodium salt first extracted from seaweed by Japanese scientists in 1908**: Jordan Sand, "A Short History of MSG: Good Science, Bad Science, and Taste Cultures," *Gastronomica: The Journal of Critical Food Studies* 5.4 (2005): 38–49.

2. **The MSG scare began on April 4, 1968**: Ian Mosby, "'That Won-Ton Soup Headache': The Chinese Restaurant Syndrome, MSG and the Making of American Food, 1968–1980," *Social History of Medicine* 22 1 (2009): 133–51. My discussion of MSG draws extensively on Mosby's excellent article.

2. **The cause is obscure**: R. H. M. Kwok, "Chinese-Restaurant Syndrome," *New England Journal of Medicine* 278 (1968): 796. The letter was titled by an editor, not Dr. Kwok.

2. **In May, the journal printed no less than ten of these letters**: Correspondence, *New England Journal of Medicine* 278 (1968): 1122–24.

3. **the *New York Times* ran an article**: R. D. Lyons, "Chinese Restaurant Syndrome Puzzles Doctors," *New York Times*, May 19, 1968. Cited in Mosby.

3. **the prestigious journal *Nature* published research**: P. L. Morselli and S. Garattini, "Monosodium Glutamate and the Chinese Restaurant Syndrome," *Nature* (1970): 611–12. Cited in Mosby.

3. **sought out a young lawyer-advocate named Ralph Nader**: Mosby.

3. **Gerber, Heinz, and Squibb Beech–Nut caved to enormous public pressure**: Ibid.

3. **the National Research Council ruled that MSG was "fit for human consumption but not necessarily by infants"**: Ibid.

4. **clinical trials strongly suggested that MSG did not produce symptoms**: See L. Tarasoff and M. F. Kelly, "Monosodium L-Glutamate: A Double-Blind Study and Review," *Food and Chemical Toxicology* 31.12 (1993): 1019–35. See also Raif S. Geha, et al., "Review of Alleged Reaction to Monosodium Glutamate and Outcome of a Multicenter Double-Blind Placebo-Controlled Study," *Journal of Nutrition* 130.4 (2000): 1058S–1062S. For a literature review, see Matthew Freeman, "Reconsidering the Effects of Monosodium Glutamate: A Literature Review," *Journal of the American Academy of Nurse Practitioners* 18.10 (2006): 482–86.

4. **the rarity of the MSG symptom complex**: Dean D. Metcalfe, et al., eds., *Food Allergy: Adverse Reaction to Foods and Food Additives* (New York: John Wiley & Sons, 2013), 378.

4. **Is MSG Misunderstood?**: Joe Donatelli, "Is MSG (Monosodium Glutamate) Misunderstood?," June 30, 2014, http://www.livestrong.com/article/1011122-msg-monosodium-glutamate-misunderstood.

7. **featuring hyperbolic headlines like this one**: Carol Kleiman, "Chinese Food Make You Crazy? MSG is No. 1 Suspect," *Chicago Tribune*, October 29, 1979.

7. **connected MSG to the following ills**: George R. Schwartz, *In Bad Taste: The MSG Syndrome: How Living without MSG Can Reduce Headache, Depression and Asthma, and Help You Get Control of Your Life* (Santa Fe, NM: Health Press, 1988).

7. **cutting-edge synthesis**: Russell L. Blaylock, *Excitotoxins: The Taste That Kills* (Santa Fe, NM: Health Press, 1996), xiii.

7. **"seen as a landmark work" and "a marker of our time"**: Ibid., xv.

7. **license to treat patients was suspended in 2006**: Schwartz was actually prescribing narcotics and amphetamines to treat a delusional disease called Morgellons. Morgellons sufferers believe they are infested with insects or parasites that cause skin lesions to sprout strange fibers. See Seth Mnookin, *The Panic Virus: A True Story of Medicine, Science, and Fear* (New York: Simon & Schuster, 2011), 90.

8. **Nutrition and the Illuminati Agenda**: "Dr. Russell Blaylock—Nutrition and the Illuminati Agenda," YouTube video, 48:36, posted by RobinMFisher, July 26, 2012, https://www.youtube.com/watch?v=d1g9YWib4mk.

8. **His most recent theory about our health problems singles out "chemtrails"**: "What Chemtrails Are Doing to Your Brain—Neurosurgeon Dr. Russell Blaylock Reveals Shocking Facts," YouTube video, 50:13, posted by Russell Blaylock, MD, April 7, 2013, https://www.youtube.com/watch?v=X3lW-TGGlk0.

8. ***60 Minutes* actually featured Schwartz in a 1991 segment**: Robert Pratt, "'60 Minutes' Report on MSG Triggers More Debate," *Chicago Tribune*, November 7, 1991.

8. **unwarranted panic among consumers**: Ibid.

9. **summarized the consensus yet again in a short video**: The American Chemical Society, "Is MSG Bad for You? Debunking a Long-Running Food Myth," August 25, 2014, http://www.acs.org/content/acs/en/pressroom/newsreleases/2014/august/is-msg-bad-for-you-debunking-a-long-running-food-myth-video.html.

9. **One article for the Huffington Post**: Joseph Mercola, "MSG: Is This Silent Killer Lurking in Your Kitchen Cabinets?," May 16, 2010, http://www.huffingtonpost.com/dr-mercola/msg-is-this-silent-killer_b_491502.html.

9. **chronic MSG ingestion by children may be one reason behind the nation's falling test scores**: Barbara L. Minton, "Consuming Common Food Additive MSG Increases Risk of Weight Gain," January 19, 2009, Written for NaturalNews.com. http://www.naturalnews.com/025353_msg_food_brain.html.

CHAPTER ONE

12. **the grain-free monks of ancient China**: Robert Ford Campany, "The Meanings of Cuisines of Transcendence in Late Classical and Early Medieval China," *T'oung Pao* (2005): 1–57. My discussion of the grain-free monks is completely indebted to Campany's work.

12. **so-called five grains**: Sometimes the five grains included wheat. See Campany, 25, for an extended discussion.

12. **the founders of Daoism**: The history of Daoism is controversial, and some scholars, including Campany, do not refer to these early practitioners as Daoists. For the sake of simplicity, I do. See Campany, 6.

12. **the scissors that cut off life**: "Les ciseaux qui coupent la vie." Jean Lévi, "L'abstinence des céréales chez les taoïstes," *Études chinoises* 1 (1982): 3–47. Lévi describes as literally demonizing grains: "une veritable mythologie démoniaque."

13. **the ability to fly *and* teleport**: Campany, 40.

13. **Plenty of them doubted accounts of flying alchemists who never got sick**: See, for instance, Wang Chong's skepticism in the *Lunheng,* described in Lévi, 5.

13. **represented rejection of modern culture**: See Campany, 51.

13. **Daoist taboos shifted from the five grains to meat and blood**: Ibid.

14. **food-based insults collected by anthropologists**: Frederick J. Simoons, *Eat Not This Flesh: Food Avoidances from Prehistory to the Present* (University of Wisconsin Press, 1994), 319–20.

16. **language of science doesn't guarantee access to the insights of science**: A classic example, described by cancer epidemiologist Geoffrey Kabat, is the perceived connection between cancer and exposure to irradiated food. Irradiation is a genuine scientific word. But, as Kabat points out in his book *Hyping Health Risks,* while scientists rate food irradiation as "low risk" and "acceptable," the public rates it as "moderate to high risk." Irradiation = unnatural = bad. Geoffrey C. Kabat, *Hyping Health Risks: Environmental Hazards in Daily Life and the Science of Epidemiology* (New York: Columbia University Press, 2011), 7.

17. **an iconic *Time* magazine cover**: *Time,* March 26, 1984.

17. **All red meat is risky, a study finds**: *Los Angeles Times,* LATExtra, March 13, 2012, http://articles.latimes.com/2012/mar/13/health/la-he-red-meat-20120313.

17. **being . . . demonized**: "Saturated Fat Heart Disease 'Myth,'" October 22, 2013, BBC Health News, http://www.bbc.com/news/health-24625808.

17. **"Longer Lives for Obese Mice"**: Apparently there is a feud between Nicholas Wade and Nicholas Bakalar about the effectiveness of resveratrol. Nicholas Wade, "Longer Lives for Obese Mice, With Hope for Humans of All Sizes," *New York Times*, August 19, 2011. This article is about new drugs that "mimic resveratrol—the trace ingredient of red wine."

17. **"Limits to Resveratrol as Metabolism Aid"**: Nicholas Bakalar, "Patterns: Limits to Resveratrol as a Metabolism Aid," *New York Times*, November 6, 2012.

17. **"New Optimism on Resveratrol"**: Nicholas Wade, "Nutrition: New Optimism on Resveratrol," *New York Times*, March 12, 2013.

17. **"Wine Ingredient May Have Few Health Benefits"**: Nicholas Bakalar, "Wine Ingredient May Have Few Health Benefits," *New York Times*, "Well Blog," May 15, 2014, http://well.blogs.nytimes.com/2014/05/15/wine-ingredient-may-have-few-health-benefits.

17. *Vogue* **magazine quotes Paleo guru Loren Cordain**: Petronella Ravenshear, "Lifting the Lid On Superfoods," *Vogue*, April 8, 2014, http://www.vogue.co.uk/news/2014/04/08/foods-of-the-gods.

18. **Why Most Published Research Findings Are False**: John P. A. Ioannidis, "Why Most Published Research Findings Are False," *PLoS Medicine* 2.8 (2005): e124.

19. **News outlets and TV shows tout his approach**: "Dr. Oz Show—The New Science of Reversing Aging," posted on Ornish's website, http://ornishspectrum.com/video/dr-oz-show-the-new-science-of-reversing-aging. See also "Dr. Oz and Dean Ornish: New Diet Science Reverses Aging from Eithin," Examiner.com, July 22, 2013, http://www.examiner.com/article/dr-oz-and-dean-ornish-new-diet-science-reverses-aging-from-within.

20. **health guru Horace Fletcher popularized his theory of mastication**: James C. Whorton, *Crusaders for Fitness: The History of American Health Reformers* (Princeton, NJ: Princeton University Press, 1982). The account of Fletcher draws on Whorton's research.

20. **no more odor than a hot biscuit**: Ibid., 178.

20. **but among those who followed it were**: Sander L. Gilman, *Diets and Dieting: A Cultural Encyclopedia* (New York: Routledge, 2008), 101.

21. **"low-hanging fruit" like "smoking and lung cancer"**: Geoffrey C. Kabat, *Hyping Health Risks: Environmental Hazards in Daily Life and the Science of Epidemiology* (New York: Columbia University Press, 2008), 5.

21. **national eating disorder**: Michael Pollan, "Our National Eating Disorder," *New York Times Magazine*, October 17, 2004.

22. **Worrying about food is not good for you**: Rozin said this to me in an interview, and a very similar quote appears in Pollan's article.

CHAPTER 2

24. **Research suggests that almost one in a hundred Americans**: "Celiac Disease: Fast Facts," National Foundation for Celiac Awareness, http://www.celiaccentral.org/celiac-disease/facts-and-figures.

24. **usually joint pain, fatigue, "foggy mind," or numbness of their extremities**: Alessio Fasano, ed., *A Clinical Guide to Gluten-Related Disorders* (Philadelphia: Wolters Kluwer/Lippincott Williams & Wilkins, 2014), 43.

25. **has grown to around $4 billion, and is projected to reach nearly $7 billion by 2019**: Markets and Markets, "Gluten-Free Products Market by Type, Sales Channel & Geography—

Global Trends & Forecasts to 2019," report summary, http://www.marketsandmarkets.com/Market-Reports/gluten-free-products-market-738.html.

25. **gluten sensitivity in Irish setters**: A. Verlinden, Myriam Hesta, Sam Millet, and G. P. J. Janssens, "Food Allergy in Dogs and Cats: A Review," *Critical Reviews in Food Science and Nutrition* 46.3 (2006): 259–73.

25. **2008 study of two large-chain general grocery stores**: Laci Stevens and Mohsin Rashid, "Gluten-Free and Regular Foods: A Cost Comparison," *Canadian Journal of Dietetic Practice and Research* 69.3 (2008): 147–50.

26. **Increased estrogen, breast cancer, man boobs**: William Davis, *Wheat Belly: Lose the Wheat, Lose the Weight, and Find Your Path Back to Health* (city TK: Rodale, 2011), 65.

26. **Is your cell phone frying your brain**: David Perlmutter and Carol Colman, *The Better Brain Book* (New York: Penguin, 2005), 154. This book also has a section on excitotoxins.

26. **so is your clock radio**: Ibid., 11.

26. **Raise IQ by up to 30 points and turn on your child's smart genes**: Carol Colman and David Perlmutter, *Raise a Smarter Child by Kindergarten: Raise IQ by up to 30 Points and Turn on Your Child's Smart Genes* (New York: Harmony Reprint, Random House LLC, 2008).

26. **Then there are the websites**: http://www.drperlmutter.com, http://www.wheatbelly-blog.com, and http://www.cureality.com.

28. **As one commenter writes breathlessly on Perlmutter's website**: http://www.drperlmutter.com/good-true, Posted by "RiRi Ray," Retrieved October 25, 2014.

29. **it is not a healthier diet for those who don't need it**: Kenneth Chang, "Gluten-Free, Whether You Need It or Not," *New York Times,* February 5, 2013.

29. **are following a fad, essentially**: Ibid.

29. **embarking on treatment, which can be burdensome to follow and adds significantly to the cost of living**: *A Clinical Guide*, 72.

29. **particularly controversial**: Ibid., xii.

29. **fantasies**: Ibid.

30. **cannot be entirely explained by a placebo effect**: Ibid., 43.

30. **irritable bowel–like symptoms of gluten sensitivity were more frequent**: Ibid.

30. **no effects of gluten in patients with self-reported non-celiac gluten sensitivity**: Jessica R. Biesiekierski, Simone L. Peters, Evan D. Newnham, Ourania Rosella, Jane G. Muir, and Peter R. Gibson, "No Effects of Gluten in Patients with Self-Reported Non-Celiac Gluten Sensitivity after Dietary Reduction of Fermentable, Poorly Absorbed, Short-Chain Carbohydrates," *Gastroenterology* 145.2 (2013): 320–28.

32. **contribute to the development of eating disorders**: Though it is not included in the DSM-V, the condition known as "orthorexia nervosa" (fixation on righteous eating) refers to eating disorders that result from obsessive attention to the type and quality of food. Steven Bratman and David Knight. *Health Food Junkies: Orthorexia Nervosa; Overcoming the Obsession with Healthful Eating* (New York: Broadway, 2001). For a recent case study and discussion: Ryan M. Moroze, Thomas M. Dunn, J. Craig Holland, Joel Yager, and Philippe Weintraub, "Microthinking about Micronutrients: A Case of Transition from Obsessions about Healthy Eating to Near-Fatal 'Orthorexia Nervosa' and Proposed Diagnostic Criteria," *Psychosomatics* (2014).

33. **cure rate of over 90 percent**: Andrew Pollack, "Gilead's Hepatitis C Drug Wins F.D.A. Approval," *New York Times,* October 11, 2014.

33. **son of actor Christopher Reeve announced a huge advance in the treatment of spinal injury**: Sharon Cotliar, "Christopher Reeve's Son Gives First Look at Amazing Progress in Spinal Cord Injury Research," *People Magazine*, October 9, 2014, http://www.people.com/article/christopher-reeve-spinal-cord-injury-breakthrough.

34. **means "sickness of the belly" in Greek**: Gee took this name from the Greek physician Aretaeus, who had described the condition in the first century CE. Samuel Gee, "On the Coeliac Affection," *St. Bartholomew's Hospital Reports*, 1888, 24, 17.

34. **The course of the disease is always slow**: Samuel Gee, "On the Coeliac Affection," *St. Bartholomew's Hospital Reports*, 1888, 24, 19.

34. **Gee could only speculate**: "The causes of the disease are obscure." Ibid., 18.

34. **preferring "asses' milk," "bread cut thin and well toasted on both sides"**: Ibid., 21.

35. **1939 British review of seventy-three cases**: Christopher Hardwick, "Prognosis in Coeliac Disease: A Review of Seventy-Three Cases," *Archives of Disease in Childhood* 14.80 (1939): 279–94.

35. **after attending a meeting of pediatricians in 1932**: G. P. van Berge-Henegouwen and C. J. Mulder, "Pioneer in the Gluten Free Diet: Willem-Karel Dicke 1905–1962, over 50 Years of Gluten Free Diet," *Gut* 34.11 (1993): 1473.

35. **I give a simple diet**: Ibid., 1474.

35. **the end of World War II provided additional evidence to confirm it**: Ibid., 1473.

35–6. **British physician Margot Shiner pioneered the use of intestinal biopsy capsules**: Emily K. Abel, "The Rise and Fall of Celiac Disease in the United States," *Journal of the History of Medicine and Allied Sciences* 65.1 (2010): 81–105. Much of this history depends on Abel's work. I am also grateful for the time she gave me in interviews to discuss the difficulty inherent in contested illness, which shaped the conclusion of this chapter.

36. **which he first detailed in a 1924 article**: Sidney Hass, "The Value of the Banana in the Treatment of Celiac Disease," *Archives of Pediatrics & Adolescent Medicine* 28.4 (1924): 421. Originally for *American Journal of Diseases of Children*. See Abel.

36. **United Fruit Company mounted an aggressive advertising campaign**: The following discussion draws heavily on Abel's article.

36. **This fruit is sealed by nature in practically germ-free and germ-proof packages**: Anon., *Food Value of the Banana: Opinion of Leading Medical and Scientific Authorities* (Boston: United Fruit, 1917), In *Food Value*, 20. Cited in Abel.

36. **Numerous dietitians testified to their curative powers**: Abel, 95–96.

36. **Of ten children treated, eight experienced dramatic symptom remission and dramatically increased height and weight**: Hass, "Value of the Banana," 421.

37. **strikingly transformed children**: Abel is clearly somewhat skeptical of Haas's reports. As she notes, the inclusion of photos and charts "lent a scientific aura to his claims." The same could be said of more recent diet books.

37. **capable of hydrolyzing**: Sidney V. Haas, "Powdered Ripe Banana in Infant Feeding," *Archives of Pediatrics* 48 (1931): 249. Cited in Abel.

37. **At Johns Hopkins, Dr. George Harrop tried it on diabetics**: Harrop was at Johns Hopkins at the same time as another important celiac researcher named John Howland, who was America's first full-time professor of pediatrics and head of the department of pediatrics. Howland was an early advocate of treating CD with a diet that included milk. There can be little

doubt that Harrop would have been familiar with the use of milk and bananas in treating celiac when he undertook his studies of diabetics.

37. **Harrop published his results in 1934**: George A. Harrop, "A Milk and Banana Diet for the Treatment of Obesity," *Journal of the American Medical Association* 102.24 (1934): 2003–5. Both Harrop and Haas emphasized the satiety provided by bananas.

37. **One Milwaukee newspaper reported**: "Reducing on a Banana-Milk Diet Brings Warning From Medical Men," *Milwaukee Journal*, May 3, 1934.

37. **will result in dramatic weight loss, but may also make you irritable**: Erin Monahan, "Banana and Milk Diet," August 16, 2013, http://www.livestrong.com/article/292271-banana-milk-diet. To be fair, Livestrong.com has another article condemning the diet: http://www.livestrong.com/article/474308-bananas-only-diet.

37–8. **like advertisements of the United Fruit Company**: John Lovett Morse, "Progress in Pediatrics," *New England Journal of Medicine* 204.13 (1931): 668–75. Cited in Abel.

38. **Bananas Help Ill Child**: "New Vaccine Held Rheumatism Check; Bananas Help Ill Child," *New York Times*, May 12, 1932. Cited in Abel.

38. *Newsweek* **and the** *New York Times* **described the odyssey of mothers**: "24 Bananas for Baby, Ill of Rare Ailment, Are Located after Police Join Frantic Hunt," *New York Times*, July 31, 1942, 17. "Banana Priorities," *Newsweek*, August 10, 1942, 20, 56–57. Cited in Abel.

38. **doing all that is possible to meet the situation**: Sidney V. Haas, "To the Editor," *New York Times*, August 4, 1942. Cited in Abel.

38. **begin feeding the baby banana at the age of four or five weeks instead of four or five months**: William Brady, "Mothers Making Baby Book Obselete," *Milwaukee Sentinel*, October 1, 1959, 11.

38. **started her three babies on banana when they were about two weeks old**: Ibid.

39. **cure which is permanent without relapse**: Sidney Haas, "Celiac Disease," *New York State Journal of Medicine* 63 (1963): 1346. Cited in Abel.

39. **Americans authored only 1 percent of research articles**: Alessio Fasano, "Where Have All the American Celiacs Gone?," *Acta Paediatrica* 85.s412 (1996): 20–24. Cited in Abel.

39. **There were no mentions of the disease in newspapers or magazines**: Abel, 103.

40. **In 1955, Judy began suffering from severe chronic intestinal distress**: "About the Author," http://www.breakingtheviciouscycle.info/p/about-the-author. The following narrative follows the About the Author section of the website.

40. **She accused doctors of being attracted to Dicke's approach because of intellectual laziness**: Elaine Gottschall, "Whatever Happened to the Cure for Coeliac Disease?," *Nutritional Therapy Today* 7.1 (1997): 8–11. Gottschall writes that accepting a gluten-free treatment for CD was appealing because it meant there would be "no need to delve into food biochemistry and ask why gluten-containing foods such as corn would be considered permissible . . . "

40. **earning a bachelor's degree in biology and a master's degree in nutritional biochemistry and cellular biology**: "About the Author," http://www.breakingtheviciouscycle.info/p/about-the-author.

41. **can truly "cure" CD**: In "Whatever Happened to the Cure for Coeliac Disease?," Gottschall writes, "The Specific Carbohydrate Diet has been shown to completely cure most cases of coeliac disease if followed for at least one year."

41. **as well as a variety of other disorders**: http://www.breakingtheviciouscycle.info/home.

41. **adds a chapter on autism**: http://www.breakingtheviciouscycle.info/p/scd-autism.

41. **The Specific Carbohydrate Diet is biologically correct**: http://www.breakingthe viciouscycle.info/p/beginners-guide.

42. **Dr. James Braly and Ron Hoggan published *Dangerous Grains***: James Braly and Ron Hoggan, *Dangerous Grains: Why Gluten Cereal Grains May Be Hazardous to Your Health* (New York: Penguin, 2002).

42. **look and act just like . . . morphine**: Ibid., 109.

42. **His September 2014 LinkedIn profile lists him**: http://www.linkedin.com/pub/james-braly-md/34/90/225.

42. **once located in Tijuana, Mexico**: "Ask the Doctor," installment 34, hosted by James Braly, http://www.stemcellpioneers.com/showthread.php?3760-Installment-34-Ask-the-Doctor-hosted-by-Dr-James-Braly.

42. **emotional, picky, fussy, attention-seeking, and a hypochondriac**: *Dangerous Grains*, xvii.

43. **Jack refused to listen**: Ibid., xix. Hoggan told me this story in great detail during our interview. After the interview was done, he became suspicious and accused me of manipulating him into giving information that he didn't want to give. I attempted to contact him after he made the accusations and failed. I have made an effort not to include details of his personal life that he disclosed to me, and to focus only on what is publicly available.

43. **months of depression, lethargy, and abdominal pain**: Ibid., xx.

43. **high prevalence of undiagnosed CD in sufferers of fibromyalgia**: Bruce Taubman, Peter Mamula, and David D. Sherry, "Prevalence of Asymptomatic Celiac Disease in Children with Fibromyalgia: A Pilot Study," *Pediatric Rheumatology* 2011, 9:11.

43. **irritable bowel syndrome**: David S. Sanders, Martyn J. Carter, David P. Hurlstone, Alison Pearce, Anthony Milford Ward, Mark E. McAlindon, and Alan J. Lobo, "Association of Adult Coeliac Disease with Irritable Bowel Syndrome: A Case-Control Study in Patients Fulfilling ROME II Criteria Referred to Secondary Care," *The Lancet* 358.9292 (2001): 1504–8.

43. **diabetes**: T. Not, A. Tommasini, G. Tonini, E. Buratti, M. Pocecco, C. Tortul, M. Valussi, et al., "Undiagnosed Coeliac Disease and Risk of Autoimmune Disorders in Subjects with Type I Diabetes Mellitus," *Diabetologia* 44.2 (2001): 151–55.

43. **atopic eczema, and other related conditions**: D. Zauli, A. Grassi, A. Granito, S. Foderaro, L. De Franceschi, G. Ballardini, F. B. Bianchi, and U. Volta, "Prevalence of Silent Coeliac Disease in Atopics," *Digestive and Liver Disease* 32.9 (2000): 775–79.

44. **particularly among sufferers of chronic health problems**: Personal interview, Ron Hoggan. He told me that online chat rooms were especially popular for spreading the word about his book.

44. **University of Google**: Jenny McCarthy, *Louder Than Words: A Mother's Journey in Healing Autism* (New York: Penguin, 2007), 166.

45. **Milder forms of celiac disease, referred to as 'gluten sensitivity,' affect about 15 percent of the population**: Joseph Mercola. *The No-Grain Diet: Conquer Carbohydrate Addiction and Stay Slim for Life* (New York: Penguin, 2004), 27.

45. **Unlike our grandparents**: Ibid., 149.

45. **beneficial for most**: Elisabeth Hasselbeck, *The G-Free Diet: A Gluten-Free Survival Guide* (New York: Center Street, 2011), 192. Dr. Peter Green actually wrote the foreword to the book, though he disagrees with Hasselbeck's position, http://glutendude.com/celebrities/elizabeth-hasselbeck-or-dr-peter-green.

45. **would still choose to be G-free**: Ibid., 183.

45. **Jennifer Aniston went gluten-free in 2010**: http://www.thedailybeast.com/galleries/2010/08/01/gluten-free-stars.html.

45. **baby-food diet**: http://www.huffingtonpost.com/2010/05/05/jennifer-aniston-put-on--b_n_564484.html.

45. **everyone should try no gluten for a week!**: https://twitter.com/MileyCyrus/status/189211162808827905.

46. **studies have shown that people respond well to fake versions of these interventions**: Karolina Wartolowska, Andrew Judge, Sally Hopewell, Gary S. Collins, Benjamin JF Dean, Ines Rombach, David Brindley, Julian Savulescu, David J. Beard, and Andrew J. Carr, "Use of Placebo Controls in the Evaluation of Surgery: Systematic Review," *BMJ: British Medical Journal* 348 (2014). David Colquhoun and Steven P. Novella, "Acupuncture Is Theatrical Placebo," *Anesthesia & Analgesia* 116.6 (2013): 1360–63.

46. **The nocebo effect is the placebo effect in reverse**: Robert A. Hahn, "The Nocebo Phenomenon: Concept, Evidence, and Implications for Public Health," *Preventive Medicine* 26.5 (1997): 607–11.

47. **One 2009 study of lactose found that fourteen out of fifty-four patients**: Piero Vernia, Mauro Di Camillo, Tiziana Foglietta, Veronica E. Avallone, and Aurora De Carolis, "Diagnosis of Lactose Intolerance and the 'Nocebo' Effect: The Role of Negative Expectations," *Digestive and Liver Disease* 42.9 (2010): 616–19.

47. **observed in the studies of gluten sensitivity out of Monash University**: "A high nocebo response was found regardless of known background dietary triggers . . . " Biesierkski et al., "No effects of gluten," 2013.

47. **in many circumstances non-celiac gluten sensitivity is an imaginary ailment**: Umberto Volta, Giacomo Caio, Francesco Tovoli, and Roberto De Giorgio, "Non-Celiac Gluten Sensitivity: Questions Still to Be Answered Despite Increasing Awareness, *Cellular & Molecular Immunology* 10.5 (2013): 386.

47. **placebo effects increase when the treatment is complicated, branded, and expensive**: A. Branthwaite and P. Cooper, clinical research edition, "Analgesic Effects of Branding in Treatment of Headaches," *British Medical Journal* 282.6276 (1981): 1576. Rebecca L. Waber, Baba Shiv, and Ziv Carmon, "Commercial Features of Placebo and Therapeutic," *JAMA* 299.9 (2008): 1016–17. Ted J. Kaptchuk, William B. Stason, Roger B. Davis, Anna RT Legedza, Rosa N. Schnyer, Catherine E. Kerr, David A. Stone, Bong Hyun Nam, Irving Kirsch, and Rose H. Goldman, "Sham Device v Inert Pill: Randomised Controlled Trial of Two Placebo Treatments," *BMJ* 332.7538 (2006): 391–97.

48. **for their extraordinary efforts:** Recent research, long overdue, is beginning to support the use of Gottschall's Specific Carbohydrate Diet for managing Crohn's and ulcerative colitis, though much more is needed to determine why it might work, for whom, and for how long—as well as to determine potential drawbacks or side effects. However, this promising research does not confirm that we should ignore the consensus of modern medicine and trust

anti-establishment diet gurus. Quite the opposite: it shows that when people like Gottschall talk overconfidently (and falsely) about "curing" celiac disease or autism they run the risk of alienating the very researchers who can help them prove the more moderate efficacy of their chosen dietary practice. This does an enormous disservice to the sufferers who stand to benefit from that research, making it difficult to distinguish genuinely potential treatments from quack panaceas. See, for instance: Stanley A. Cohen, et al., "Clinical and Mucosal Improvement with the Specific Carbohydrate Diet in Pediatric Crohn's Disease: A Prospective Pilot Study," *Journal of Pediatric Gastroenterology and Nutrition* (2014).

48. **began on June 8, 1999, at a small school in Bornem, Belgium**: Benoit Nemery, Benjamin Fischler, Marc Boogaerts, Dominique Lison, and Jan Willems, "The Coca-Cola Incident in Belgium, June 1999," *Food and Chemical Toxicology* 40.11 (2002): 1657–67. My account is based on this extremely detailed article.

49. **all suspected carcinogens**: Jouko Tuomisto and Jouni T. Tuomisto, "Is the Fear of Dioxin Cancer More Harmful Than Dioxin?," *Toxicology Letters* 210.3 (2012): 338–44.

49. **The dioxin crisis, therefore, combined a number of factors that are known to influence risk perception greatly**: "The Coca-Cola Incident," 2.2.

50. **The remarkable consistency of the reported complaints**: Benoit Nemery, Benjamin Fischler, Marc Boogaerts, and Dominique Lison, "Dioxins, Coca-Cola, and Mass Sociogenic Illness in Belgium," *The Lancet* 347.9172 (1999): 77.

50. **who believed they were possessed by demons would imitate animals**: Robert E. Bartholomew and Simon Wessely, "Protean Nature of Mass Sociogenic Illness: From Possessed Nuns to Chemical and Biological Terrorism Fears," *British Journal of Psychiatry* 180.4 (2002): 300–306.

50. **produced chills, headaches, nausea, and breathlessness among students at a Singapore high school**: Ibid.

50. **the same occurred in 1998 at a high school in Tennessee**: Timothy F. Jones, Allen S. Craig, Debbie Hoy, Elaine W. Gunter, David L. Ashley, Dana B. Barr, John W. Brock, and William Schaffner, "Mass Psychogenic Illness Attributed to Toxic Exposure at a High School," *New England Journal of Medicine* 342.2 (2000): 96–100.

50. **The syndrome is widely publicized in English-speaking countries**: See Ketan Joshi, "Diseases That Speak English," blog post, October 6, 2012, http://etwasluft.blogspot.com/2012/10/diseases-that-speak-english.html. See also Simon Chapman, "Wind turbine syndrome: a classic 'communicated' disease," July 19, 2012, http://theconversation.com/wind-turbine-syndrome-a-classic-communicated-disease-8318.

50. **To study the mechanism of wind turbine syndrome**: Fiona Crichton, George Dodd, Gian Schmid, Greg Gamble, and Keith J. Petrie, "Can Expectations Produce Symptoms from Infrasound Associated with Wind Turbines?," *Health Psychology* 33.4 (2014): 360.

51. **His 2008 opinion piece for the *British Medical Journal***: Nicholas A. Christakis, "This Allergies Hysteria Is Just Nuts," *BMJ: British Medical Journal* 337.7683 (2008): 1384. See also Miranda R. Waggoner, "Parsing the Peanut Panic: The Social Life of a Contested Food Allergy Epidemic," *Social Science & Medicine* 90 (2013): 49–55.

53. **Lifetime prevalence estimates in Americans of anorexia**: James I. Hudson, Eva Hiripi, Harrison G. Pope Jr., and Ronald C. Kessler, "The Prevalence and Correlates of Eating Disorders in the National Comorbidity Survey Replication," *Biological Psychiatry* 61.3 (2007): 348–58.

53. **mortality rate of at least 4 percent**: http://www.anad.org/get-information/about-eating-disorders/eating-disorders-statistics.

53. **ten times more yearly deaths from anorexia**: According to Meredith Broussard, most estimates of food allergy deaths are exaggerated. See her "Everyone's Gone Nuts," *Harper's*, January 2008. Broussard puts the number of annual food deaths at around 12, compared with a very conservative estimate of 145 annual deaths from anorexia *alone*. See Paul L. Hewitt, Stanley Coren, and G. D. Steel, "Death from Anorexia Nervosa: Age Span and Sex Differences," *Aging & Mental Health* 5.1 (2001): 41–46.

53. **Gluten confirmed to cause serious weight gain**: http://www.naturalnews.com/038699_gluten_weight_gain_wheat_belly.html.

53. **Three Hidden Ways That Wheat Makes You Fat**: Dr. Mark Hyman peppers his terrifyingly titled article with great turns of phrase: "wheat weaves its misery," "tsunami of chronic illness," "FrankenFoods." He also includes the obligatory gesture to grandparents: "This is not the wheat your great-grandmother used to bake her bread," http://www.huffingtonpost.com/dr-mark-hyman/wheat-gluten_b_1274872.html.

56. **In my case**: Amy Kubal, "Coming Out," blog post, February 12, 2014, http://robbwolf.com/2014/02/12/coming-out. Robb Wolf, the curator of a wildly popular Paleo website and one of Paleo's most revered gurus, deserves praise for posting Amy's piece. Hopefully it will serve to inspire serious soul-searching in the community of elimination dieters.

57. **has spent much of his career criticizing how everyday symptoms**: Nortin M. Hadler, *Worried Sick: A Prescription for Health in an Overtreated America* (University of North Carolina Press, 2012). Hadler is not the first to title a book about these problems "worried sick." For a dated version of similar arguments, see Arthur J. Barsky, *Worried Sick: Our Troubled Quest for Wellness* (New York: Little, Brown and Co, 1988).

58. **A firm public message that certain symptoms are probably psychological**: Simon Wessely, "Responding to Mass Psychogenic Illness," *New England Journal of Medicine* 342.2 (2000): 129–30.

58. **routinely identified as hysteria**: Louis R. Caplan and Theodore Nadelson. "Multiple Sclerosis and Hysteria: Lessons Learned from Their Association," *JAMA* 243.23 (1980): 2418–21.

59. **"[They] would tell of their own devastating health problems**: Harvey A. Levenstein, *Revolution at the Table: The Transformation of the American Diet* (University of California Press, 1988), 86. Also cited in Abel.

59. **regimen in a recent radio debate**: Davis debated Tim Caufield, professor of health law and science policy and author of *The Cure For Everything: Untangling the Twisted Messages About Health, Fitness, and Happiness*, http://www.cbc.ca/q/blog/2013/02/07/are-wheat-free-diets-a-fad; Matthew Chang and Peter H. R. Green, "Genetic Testing Before Serologic Screening in Relatives of Patients with Celiac Disease as a Cost Containment Method, *Journal of Clinical Gastroenterology* 43.1 (2009): 43–50.

60. **calls on all people who suspect gluten sensitivity to go to a doctor and get tested**: http://www.oregonlive.com/living/index.ssf/2012/02/focus_on_gluten_q_a_with_celia.html. See also: Peter H. R. Green and Rory Jones, *Celiac Disease: A Hidden Epidemic* (New York: Collins, 2006).

61. **as Dr. Joseph Murray of the Mayo Clinic put it in an interview**: Jane Brody, "When Gluten Sensitivity Isn't Celiac Disease," *New York Times*, October 6, 2014, http://well.blogs.nytimes.com/2014/10/06/when-gluten-sensitivity-isnt-celiac-disease/?_php=true&_type=blogs&_r=0.

61. **Just ask Dr. Alessio Fasano**: Transcribed podcast from www.glutenfreeschool.com, May 20, 2014, http://www.glutenfreeschool.com/2014/05/20/alessio-fasano-gluten-freedom.

CHAPTER 3

63. **"ice-structuring proteins" cloned from Arctic fish**: Julia Moskin, "Creamy, Healthier Ice Cream? What's the Catch?," *New York Times*, July 26, 2006, http://www.nytimes.com/2006/07/26/dining/26cream.html?pagewanted=print.

63. **special batters that prevent french fries from absorbing cooking oil**: Alexandra Sifferlin, "Have It the Healthier Way: Burger King Reveals Low-Fat Satisfries," September 24, 2013, for *Time*'s online "Healthland" section, http://healthland.time.com/2013/09/24/have-it-the-healthier-way-burger-king-reveals-low-fat-satisfries.

63. **The American Heart Association advises us**: For the AHA's low-fat cooking advice, see their low-fat, low-cholesterol cookbook. *American Heart Association Low-Fat, Low-Cholesterol Cookbook: Delicious Recipes to Help Lower Your Cholesterol*, 4th ed. (New York: Clarkson Potter, 2008). They are not a fun bunch, the AHA. "If you do drink alcohol, do so in moderation. If you don't drink, don't start." Even though "moderate intake of alcohol may reduce the risk for heart disease"? Ibid., 7.

64. **will help prevent heart disease and keep off extra weight**: Ibid., 3–5.

64. **Decades of sound science**: http://www.heart.org/HEARTORG/General/Frequently-Asked-Questions-About-Saturated-Fats_UCM_463756_Article.jsp.

64. **does not mention a 2012 study published in the** *American Journal of Clinical Nutrition*: Marcia C. de Oliveira Otto, Dariush Mozaffarian, Daan Kromhout, Alain G. Bertoni, Christopher T. Sibley, David R. Jacobs, and Jennifer A. Nettleton, "Dietary Intake of Saturated Fat by Food Source and Incident Cardiovascular Disease: The Multi-Ethnic Study of Atherosclerosis," *American Journal of Clinical Nutrition* 96.2 (2012): 397–404.

64–5. **which called into question the wisdom of reducing saturated fat**: Rajiv Chowdhury, Samantha Warnakula, Setor Kunutsor, Francesca Crowe, Heather A. Ward, Laura Johnson, Oscar H. Franco, et al., "Association of Dietary, Circulating, and Supplement Fatty Acids with Coronary Risk: A Systematic Review and Meta-Analysis," *Annals of Internal Medicine* 160.6 (2014): 398–406. This study generated fierce objections, especially after the authors had to correct errors in the original article. Like most nutrition science, it proves nothing positive, but adds to the mountain of evidence that most dietary guidelines are based on legitimately contested conclusions.

65. **Danes are comparatively healthy and svelte**: http://www.noo.org.uk/NOO_about_obesity/adult_obesity/international.

65. **levied the world's first tax on saturated fat**: Marion Nestle, "World's First Fat Tax: What Will It Achieve?," *New Scientist*, October 23, 2011, http://www.newscientist.com/article/mg21228356.600-worlds-first-fat-tax-what-will-it-achieve.html#.VE1mU76przI.

65. **Let us congratulate Denmark on what could be viewed as a revolutionary experiment**: Ibid.

66. **Except the science wasn't clear**: Not even to Danish scientists at the time. See this postmortem presentation by faculty at the University of Copenhagen: https://acss.org.uk/wp-content/uploads/2014/01/5-AcSS-IAG-Seminar-3-Holm.pdf.

66. **in a sense, equivalent to mass murder**: William Borders, "New Diet Decried by Nutritionists," *New York Times*, July 7, 1965. Cited in Susan Berkowitz, *The Hundred Year Diet: America's Voracious Appetite for Losing Weight* (New York: Rodale, 2010).

66. **Taubes made a compelling case**: Gary Taubes, "The Soft Science of Dietary Fat," *Science* 291.5513 (2001): 2536–45. Gary Taubes, "What If It's All Been a Big Fat Lie?," *New York Times Magazine* 7 (2002).

67. **high-fat diets were no worse than low-fat diets**: For a recent meta-analysis of branded diets, see Bradley C. Johnston, Steve Kanters, Kristofer Bandayrel, Ping Wu, Faysal Naji, Reed A. Siemieniuk, Geoff DC Ball, et al., "Comparison of Weight Loss Among Named Diet Programs in Overweight and Obese Adults: A Meta-Analysis," *JAMA* 312.9 (2014): 923–33.

67. **Walter Willett told CNN**: http://www.cnn.com/2014/06/06/health/saturated-fat-debate.

67. **collective turn to SnackWell's cookies**: David Katz, "Is All Saturated Fat the Same?," June 15, 2011, http://www.huffingtonpost.com/david-katz-md/saturated-fat_b_875401.html.

67. **were almost certainly silly to do so**: David Katz, "Scapegoats, Saints and Saturated Fats: Old Mistakes in New Directions," October 24, 2013, http://www.huffingtonpost.com/david-katz-md/saturated-fat_b_4156320.html.

68. **We have very compelling evidence**: Katz, "Is All Saturated Fat the Same?"

68. **declares on its website**: "'Eat Butter'? The Skinny On Saturated Fat," June 19, 2014, http://blog.aicr.org/2014/06/19/eat-butter-the-skinny-on-saturated-fat.

68. **simply the way that works for you**: Freedhoff confirmed this to me in an interview. Also see this characteristically levelheaded blog post, "Atkins—the King of Diets?," March 6, 2007, http://www.weightymatters.ca/2007/03/atkins-king-of-diets.html.

69. **Aseem Malhotra stated flat-out**: Aseem Malhotra, "Saturated Fat Is Not the Major Issue," *BMJ: British Medical Journal* 347 (2013).

69. **government's advice is based on a wealth of evidence**: Sarah Boseley, "Butter and Cheese Better Than Trans-Fat Margarines, Says Heart Specialist," Guardian.com, October 23, 2013, http://www.theguardian.com/lifeandstyle/2013/oct/22/butter-cheese-saturated-fat-heart-specialist.

69. **From the analysis of the independent evidence that I have done**: Charlie Cooper, "Top Heart Doctor: Unprocessed Fatty Foods May Actually Be Good for You," Independent.com, October 23, 2013, http://www.independent.co.uk/life-style/health-and-families/health-news/top-heart-doctor-unprocessed-fatty-foods-may-actually-be-good-for-you-8897707.html.

70. **All of the ailments that have been ascribed to eating fat over the years**: Nina Teicholz, *The Big Fat Surprise: Why Butter, Meat and Cheese Belong in a Healthy Diet* (New Yourk: Simon and Schuster, 2014), 28.

71. **He scrupulously avoided any other food that might contain either sugar or starch, in particular bread, milk, sweets, beer, and potatoes**: Gary Taubes, *Good Calories, Bad Calories* (New York: Random House LLC, 2007), x.

71. **the removal, as far as possible, of all saccharine, starchy, and fatty foods**: William A. Woodbury, *How to Get Thin and How to Acquire Plumpness: A Text Book for Professional and Private Use* (G. W. Dillingham, 1915), 15.

71. **for its fattening character**: William Banting, *Letter on Corpulence, Addressed to the Public . . . with Addenda* (Harrison, 1869), 47.

72. **a quirky appetite for eating tiger penis and drinking tiger blood**: Shaojie Huang, "Businessman Guilty of Killing and Eating Tigers," Sinosphere blog for *New York Times,* June 13, 2014, http://sinosphere.blogs.nytimes.com/2014/06/13/businessman-guilty-of-killing-and-eating-tigers.

72. **the *New York Times* ran an article about dwindling tiger and rhinoceros**: Philip Shenon, "The World; Poachers 'n' Tigers 'n' Bears," *New York Times,* December 11, 1994.

72. **In the reductionist view of Chinese medical practitioners**: Ibid.

73. **Native Americans believed that eating venison made you fleet of foot**: James George Frazer, *The Golden Bough: A Study in Magic and Religion,* Accessed on Project Gutenberg, LI, Homeopathic Magic of a Flesh Diet, http://www.gutenberg.org/dirs/etext03/bough11h.htm. All of the examples are taken from this section. Frazer refers to the Mishing people of India as "the Miris of Assam."

73. **The Chinese market for tiger penis is shrinking**: William Von Hippel, Frank A. Von Hippel, Norman Chan, and Clara Cheng, "Exploring the Use of Viagra in Place of Animal and Plant Potency Products in Traditional Chinese Medicine," *Environmental Conservation* 32.3 (2005): 235–38.

74. **Writing in the second century CE, the Greek physician Galen distinguished three kinds of fat people**: Niki S. Papavramidou, Spiros T. Papavramidis, and Helen Christopoulou-Aletra, "Galen on Obesity: Etiology, Effects, and Treatment," *World Journal of Surgery* 28.6 (2004): 631–35. The information on Galen comes entirely from this article.

74. **During the early Renaissance, doctors claimed that red grapes**: Ken Albala, *Eating Right in the Renaissance* (University of California Press, 2002), 80.

74. **sympathetic magic provided the logic**: Ibid., 168.

75. **As food historian Ken Albala points out**: Ken Albala, "Weight Loss in the Age of Reason," in Christopher E. Forth and Ana Carden-Coyne, eds., *Cultures of the Abdomen: Diet, Digestion, and Fat in the Modern World* (New York: Palgrave Macmillan, 2005), 171.

75. **who locked fat patients in a box lined with electric lightbulbs**: Christopher E. Forth, "The Belly of Paris," ibid., 214.

75. **Johann Friedrich Held, the first person to define obesity according to belt size**: Albala, ibid., 175–77.

76. **Historian Lucia Dacome chronicles how British consumer society faced rising obesity rates**: "Useless and Pernicious Matter: Corpulence in Eighteenth-Century England," ibid.

76. **no Age did ever afford more Instances of Corpulency than our own**: Thomas Short, *A Discourse Concerning the Causes and Effects of Corpulency: Together with the Method for Its Prevention and Cure. By Thomas Short, MD,* J. Roberts, near the Oxford Arms in Warwick Lane, 1727, 10.

76. **wearing flannel shirts and moving from marshy areas**: Ibid, 75, 11.

76. **particularly veal, pork, bacon, lamb, and mutton, in favor of fish and fowl**: Ibid., 72. Short says that fish and fowl are "less nutritious," which means he may have had something like calorie reduction in mind when forbidding fatty meats. At the same time, he appears to think some foods are undesirable because they are less easily digested and end up staying in the body, among them vegetables and shellfish. His rationale is not entirely clear, but whatever else can be said, he certainly disapproves of fatty meat, and his only explicit recommendation is "bread of oats, rye, or barley." Not exactly low carb.

76. **Water a little acidulated with Vinegar, or Juice of Lemons**: Ibid., 73.

76. **moderate, spare**: Ibid., 72.

76. **only to the Rich, the Lazy, the Luxurious**: George Cheyne, *The English Malady, Or a Treatise of Nervous Diseases of All Kinds . . . by George Cheyne,* 1733, 28. Cited in Fredrik Albritton Jonsson, "The Physiology of Hypochondria in Eighteenth-Century Britain," ibid., 17.

76. **seeds, bread, mealy roots, and fruit**: *The English Malady*, 337.

77. **persons indulging in animal food**: William Wadd, *Cursory remarks on corpulence; or Obesity considered as a disease*, Reprint 1816, 79.

77. **strong evidence of the efficacy of vegetable diet**: Ibid., 40.

77. **rich and opulent**: Ibid., 80.

77. **without any other sustenance than the ripe sugar cane**: Ibid., 79.

77. **Of the efficacy of animal or vegetable food in the reduction of corpulency**: Ibid., 78.

78. **and the animals whom he has infected with his society**: Percy Bysshe Shelley, *A Vindication of Natural Diet*, No. 4, F. Pitman, 1886, 12.

78. **an incredible variety of distempers**: Ibid., 12.

78. **pimp for the gluttony of death**: Ibid., 26.

78. **who lived long because they practiced abstinence from animal flesh**: Ibid., 27.

78. **William Lambe used the supposed connection between obesity and animal fat to generalize about the dangers of eating meat**: William Lambe and Joel Shew, *Water and Vegetable Diet in Consumption, Scrofula, Cancer, Asthma, and Other Chronic Diseases* (Fowlers & Wells, 1854). This was the title of the American reprint. The original 1815 British edition was titled *Additional Reports on the Effects of a Peculiar Regimen in Cases of Cancer, Scrofula, Consumption, Asthma, and Other Chronic Diseases*.

79. **exceedingly fat on a diet of strong ale, "animal food," and "large quantities of butter and cheese"**: Ibid., 60.

79. **It affords no trifling grounds of suspicion against animal food**: Ibid., 73.

79. **Just as eating fat makes you fat, eating animals exacerbates your animal instincts, in turn increasing your appetite for food and sex**: Sylvester Graham, *A Defence of the Graham System of Living: Or, Remarks on Diet and Regimen. Dedicated to the Rising Generation* (W. Applegate, 1835). See, for instance, 114 ff.

79. **To support his claims, Graham dutifully collected anecdotes of vegetarian longevity**: Ibid., 25 ff.

79. **man is not provided with sharpness of fangs**: Ibid., 105.

79. **California citrus producers popularized the Hollywood Eighteen-Day Diet**: Harvey A. Levenstein, *Paradox of Plenty: A Social History of Eating in Modern America* (University of California Press, 2003), 11.

79. **from a variety of popular two-food diets**: Ibid.

79. **There was the grapefruit juice diet**: Ibid.

80. **only because the acidic pineapple would "digest" the lamb**: Berkowitz, *The Hundred Year Diet*, 34.

80. **It was a smash hit at the University of Michigan**: Ibid.

80. **The changing-American-diet story envisions the turn of the century as an idyllic era**: Taubes, *Good Calories, Bad Calories*, 10.

81. **He and his associates wrote two descriptions of a people**: Carol Nemeroff and Paul Rozin, "'You Are What You Eat': Applying the Demand-Free 'Impressions' Technique to an Unacknowledged Belief," *Ethos* 17.1 (1989): 50–69.

81. **In another study, psychologist Michael Oakes**: Michael E. Oakes, "Stereotypical Thinking about Foods and Perceived Capacity to Promote Weight Gain," *Appetite* 44.3 (2005): 317–24.

82. **To test the effects of low-fat labels on food consumption**: Brian Wansink and Pierre Chandon, "Can 'Low-Fat' Nutrition Labels Lead to Obesity?," *Journal of Marketing Research* 43.4 (2006): 605–17.

83. **UCLA sociologist Abigail Saguy has made the case that it doesn't**: Abigail C. Saguy, *What's Wrong with Fat?* (Oxford University Press, 2012).

83. **she found that a "personal responsibility frame" dominated coverage of obesity**: Ibid., 71 ff.

83. **Americans are becoming fatter because they are becoming more slothful and self-indulgent**: Ibid., 72.

83. **In a study of 620 primary care physicians in the United States**: Gary D. Foster, Thomas A. Wadden, Angela P. Makris, Duncan Davidson, Rebecca Swain Sanderson, David B. Allison, and Amy Kessler, "Primary Care Physicians' Attitudes about Obesity and Its Treatment," *Obesity Research* 11.10 (2003): 1168–77. Cited in Saguy, 74.

83. **"No one to blame" is the subtitle**: Peg Tyre, "Fighting Anorexia—No One to Blame," *Newsweek*, December 4, 2005. Cited in Saguy.

84. **In 2011, Allison and coauthors published the results of research on animal populations**: Yann C. Klimentidis, T. Mark Beasley, Hui-Yi Lin, Giulianna Murati, Gregory E. Glass, Marcus Guyton, Wendy Newton, et al., "Canaries in the Coal Mine: A Cross-Species Analysis of the Plurality of Obesity Epidemics," *Proceedings of the Royal Society B: Biological Sciences* 278.1712 (2011): 1626–32.

85. **The AHA advocates keeping total dietary fat *of any kind***: http://www.heart.org/HEARTORG/Conditions/Cholesterol/PreventionTreatmentofHighCholesterol/Know-Your-Fats_UCM_305628_Article.jsp.

85. **Harvard School of Public Health states**: http://www.hsph.harvard.edu/nutrition-source/healthy-eating-plate.

CHAPTER 4

87. **How Sweet Can Become Toxic**: http://healthland.time.com/2013/08/14/how-sweet-can-become-toxic.

88. **filmmakers provide a litany of sobering statistics on the documentary's website**: http://fedupmovie.com/#/page/about-the-issue?scrollTo=facts.

88. **it has fifty-six names**: E-mail, Fed Up Challenge Day 2.

88. **fifteen more than Satan**: The number of names is debated. Here's a handy reference to those that occur in the Bible: http://www.markbeast.com/satan/names-of-satan.htm.

89. **issued its new guidelines on sugar consumption**: "WHO opens public consultation on draft sugars guidelines," March 5, 2014. The absolute limit for sugar consumption is 10 percent of total calories, and the target is below 5 percent, http://www.who.int/mediacentre/news/notes/2014/consultation-sugar-guideline/en.

90. **One of Waters's many accomplishments is a program called Edible Schoolyard**: http://edibleschoolyard.org/our-story.

90. **what she calls the "insidious," "dishonest" culture of fast food**: Lindsey Christians, "Alice Waters Decries 'Insidious' Fast Food Culture," *Capital Times,* March 28, 2014.

90. **We're in the middle of a health epidemic**: Roberta Furger, "Middle School Students Grow Their Own Lunch," March 11, 2004, Edutopia.com, http://www.edutopia.org/garden-of-eating-middle-schoolers-grow-lunch.

90. **The opening paragraph of a 2004 ESY profile reads like Big Sugar propaganda**: Ibid.

90. **The Edible Schoolyard website even features a recipe for "Celebratory Apple Crisp"**: Kyle Cornforth, "Celebratory Apple Crisp," March 8, 2013, Accessed October 27, 2014, http://edibleschoolyard.org/node/8113.

91. **Sugar: The Bitter Truth**: Lustig's presentation has more than 5 million views, https://www.youtube.com/watch?v=dBnniua6-oM.

91. **Tobacco, alcohol, cocaine, heroin, and morphine feature as prominent analogies**: Robert H. Lustig, *Fat Chance: Beating the Odds Against Sugar, Processed Food, Obesity, and Disease* (New York: Penguin, 2012). Open to pretty much any random page and you'll see what I'm talking about.

91. **the primary reason that numbers of obese and diabetic Americans have skyrocketed in the past 30 years**: Gary Taubes, "Is Sugar Toxic?," *New York Times Magazine*, April 17, 2011.

92. **A 2013 systematic review**: Maira Bes-Rastrollo, Matthias B. Schulze, Miguel Ruiz-Canela, and Miguel A. Martinez-Gonzalez, "Financial Conflicts of Interest and Reporting Bias Regarding the Association Between Sugar-Sweetened Beverages and Weight Gain: A Systematic Review of Systematic Reviews," *PLoS Medicine* 10.12 (2013): e1001578.

92. **In a 2014 exposé, the *Washington Post***: Tom Hamburger, "'Soft Lobbying' War Between Sugar, Corn Syrup Shows New Tactics in Washington Influence," *Washington Post*, February 12, 2014.

92. **The online "about the author" section catalogs Dr. Rippe's extensive credentials**: http://www.springer.com/new+%26+forthcoming+titles+%28default%29/book/978-1-4899-8076-2?detailsPage=authorsAndEditors.

93. **Taubes and coauthor Cristin Kearns Couzens documented how Big Sugar**: G. Taubes and C. K. Couzens, "Big Sugar's Sweet Little Lies: How the Industry Kept Scientists from Asking: Does Sugar Kill?," *Mother Jones* (2012).

94. **They still do**: See, for instance, Alan Bavley and Mike McGraw, "Big Beef: Industry Fights Back Using Money, Science," *Kansas City Star*, December 11, 2012. See also the American Dairy Science Institute: http://www.adsa.org.

95. **Although the brain's reward system is complex**: Lustig, *Fat Chance*, 50.

95. **fructose delivery vehicle, similar to cigarettes**: Ibid., 197.

95. **both of whom think the food addiction model has serious shortcomings**: See the following: H. Ziauddeen and P. C. Fletcher, "Is Food Addiction a Valid and Useful Concept?," *Obesity Reviews* 14.1 (2013): 19–28. See also: Hisham Ziauddeen, I. Sadaf Farooqi, and Paul C. Fletcher, "Obesity and the Brain: How Convincing Is the Addiction Model?," *Nature Reviews Neuroscience* 13.4 (2012): 279–86.

96. **A late-2013 state-of-the-field piece in the journal *Metabolism***: Byung-Joon Ko, Kyung Hee Park, and Christos S. Mantzoros, "Diet Patterns, Adipokines, and Metabolism: Where Are We and What Is Next?," *Metabolism: Clinical and Experimental* 63.2 (2014): 168.

96–7. **anything that is extremely pleasurable, and that includes sex and sweetness, must be bad**: Paul Rozin, "Sweetness, sensuality, sin, safety, and socialization: some speculations," In *Sweetness*, pp. 99–111 (Springer London, 1987), 100.

97. **In a 1996 survey, nearly a third of Americans agreed that a diet free of sugar**: Paul Rozin, Michele Ashmore, and Maureen Markwith, "Lay American Conceptions of Nutrition: Dose Insensitivity, Categorical Thinking, Contagion, and the Monotonic Mind," *Health Psychology* 15.6 (1996): 438.

98. **describes how the '60s and '70s saw an explosion of "sucrophobia" in Britain and America**: Harvey Levenstein, *Fear of Food: A History of Why We Worry about What We Eat* (University of Chicago Press, 2012), 145 ff.

98. **National Commission on Egg Nutrition in America invited Yudkin on a media tour**: An article from the *New York Times* service, by Jean Hewitt, was published with various headlines. See "British Doctor Defends the Egg," *Eugene Register-Guard,* December 26, 1974.

98. **who refers to Yudkin as a "prophet" and himself as a "disciple" and an "acolyte"**: For "prophet" and "acolyte," see Lustig's YouTube video, "The Bitter Truth," around minute 32:00. For "disciple," see John Yudkin, *Pure, White and Deadly: How Sugar Is Killing Us and What We Can Do to Stop It* (New York: Penguin, 2013), xiv and xv.

99. **in which he blamed sugar for everything from rape to the rise of Nazism**: Jerome Irving Rodale, *Natural Health, Sugar and the Criminal Mind* (Pyramid Books, 1968).

99. **sugar addiction as "the white plague," food products as "laced with sugar," and his own habit as "the road to perdition"**: William Dufty, *Sugar Blues* (New York: Warner Books, 1975), 1, 96, and 14. For an analysis of Dufty and Yudkin as moralists, see Elizabeth Walker Mechling and Jay Mechling, "Sweet Talk: The Moral Rhetoric Against Sugar," *Communication Studies* 34.1 (1983): 19–32.

99. **"Only within the past three years," wrote Crook, "have I become aware that sugar . . . "**: William C. Crook, "An Alternate Method of Managing the Hyperactive Child," *Pediatrics* 54.5 (1974): 656.

99. **as documented by the National Institute of Mental Health**: National Institute of Mental Health, "What is Attention Deficit Hyperactivity Disorder?" Accessed October 28, 2014, http://www.nimh.nih.gov/health/publications/attention-deficit-hyperactivity-disorder/index.shtml.

100. **with the end in mind of nourishment, but rather for ease of digestion**: Sidney Mintz, "Sugar and Morality," *Morality and Health* (1997): 173–84.

100. **According to sugar historian Sidney Mintz**: Sidney Wilfred Mintz, *Sweetness and Power* (New York: Viking, 1985).

100. **sugar hath now succeeded hon[ey]**: James Hart, "The Diet of the Diseased," London: John Beale for Thomas Allot, 1633. Cited in Abbot, Elizabeth, *Sugar: A Bitterweet History* (New York: Penguin, 2010).

100. **that it, too, can rot the teeth**: William H. Bowen and Ruth A. Lawrence, "Comparison of the Cariogenicity of Cola, Honey, Cow Milk, Human Milk, and Sucrose," *Pediatrics* 116.4 (2005): 921–26.

101. **cause of many distempers**: Jonas Hanway, *A journal of eight days journey from Portsmouth to Kingston upon Thames*, H. Woodfall, 1756, ix.

101. **fantastic desires and bad habits in which nature has no part**: Ibid., 39.

101. **pernicious Foreigner, called *Sugar***: Cited in Mintz, "Sugar and Morality."

101. **Children, Hanway warned, were particularly susceptible to sugar's detrimental effects**: Hanway, *A journal*, 221.

101. **products defiled with blood**: Lowell J. Ragatz, *The Fall of the Planter Class in the British Caribbean, 1763–1833* (New York: Appleton-Century), 262. Cited in Mintz, "Sugar and Morality," 176.

102. **the selling of their little black brothers into bondage**: Ibid.

102. **African Americans chose the sweetest and saltiest solutions**: Michael Moss, *Salt Sugar Fat: How the Food Giants Hooked Us* (New York: Random House, 2013), 8.

102. **Neither *Fed Up* nor *Salt Sugar Fat* mentions that white children consume a higher proportion of their calories**: Nicholar Bakalar, "Added Sugars Pile Up on Children's Plates," *New York Times,* March 19, 2012.

102. **Neither mentions that family income is irrelevant**: Ibid.

103. **Shopkeepers like Nicholas Bayard**: Wendy A. Woloson, *Refined Tastes: Sugar, Confectionery, and Consumers in Nineteenth-Century America,* No. 1 (Johns Hopkins University Press, 2002), 47. The following discussion draws extensively on Woloson's work.

103. **Penny candy, more accessible to larger groups of younger people**: Ibid., 49.

103. **We always regard it as an ill omen**: *The Friend, A Religious and Literary Journal,* vol. VIII, 141.

104. **Whereas fruit does contain fructose, it also has inherent fiber**: 133.

104. **As Yale nutritionist Dr. David Katz points out**: David Katz, "Fructose, Fruit, and Frittering," August 2, 2013, http://www.huffingtonpost.com/david-katz-md/fructose-fruit_b_3694684.html.

105. **honey contains dozens of different substances**: Cal Orey, *The Healing Powers of Honey* (Kensington Publishing Corp., 2011), 44.

105. **"Should you eat it?" asks Sisson**: Mark Sisson, "Is Honey a Safe(r) Sweetener?" Blog post, February 8, 2012, http://www.marksdailyapple.com/is-honey-a-safer-sweetener/#axzz3HRj3oNDZ.

106. **near unanimous consensus that the biological effects of high-fructose corn syrup are essentially the same as those of honey**: For an excellent review of the evidence, see Jim Laidler, "High Fructose Corn Syrup: Tasty Toxin or Slandered Sweetener?," August 23, 2010, http://www.sciencebasedmedicine.org/high-fructose-corn-syrup.

106. **stage in the down-hill course of deception and mockery, of cowardice, cruelty, and degradation**: James W. Redfield, *Comparative Physiognomy or Resemblances between Men and Animals: Illustrated by 330 Engravings* (Redfield, 1852), 270.

106. **as, for example, the housefly, the ant that lives in the sugar-bowl**: Ibid.

107. **I'm not eager to help the corn refiners sell more of their stuff**: Tara Parker-Pope, "A New Name for High-Fructose Corn Syrup," *New York Times,* September 14, 2010.

107. **In a 2014 blog post about Fig Newtons**: Vani Hari, "The Ingredients in This Popular Snack Might Surprise You," Foodbabe.com, July 29, 2014, http://foodbabe.com/2014/07/29/fig-newtons-100-whole-grain.

107. **Five Reasons High Fructose Corn Syrup Will Kill You**: http://drhyman.com/blog/2011/05/13/5-reasons-high-fructose-corn-syrup-will-kill-you.

108. **The use of sugar is the stepping-stone to intemperance**: Redfield, 270–71. Cited in Woloson, 60.

108. **the sugar out of the bottom of his father's toddy-glass**: Cited in Woloson, 36.

108. **The appetite for alcohol and the appetite for candy are fundamentally the same**: Ibid., 62.

108. **Founding Father Benjamin Rush wrote a book**: Benjamin Rush, *Medical Inquiries and Observations upon the Diseases of the Mind* (John Grigg, 1830).

108. **The idea of addiction turned demonic possession into a physical condition**: Joseph W. Schneider, "Deviant Drinking as Disease: Alcoholism as a Social Accomplishment," *Social Problems* (1978): 361–72.

109. **Initially soda fountains were perceived as providing a clean, dainty, ladylike alternative to men's taverns**: See Woloson, 99.

109. **Myth No. 3 in the American Diabetes Association's myths section**: http://www. diabetes.org/diabetes-basics/myths.

110. **Hilariously, ice cream parlors inspired sensational tales**: See chapters 3 and 4 of Woloson.

110. **great enemy of [women's] souls**: Cited in Woloson, 138.

110. **Candies, spices, cinnamon, cloves, peppermint, and all strong essences**: John Harvey Kellogg, *Plain Facts for Old and Young* (I. F. Segner, 1882), 330.

110. **penalties which God, in his providence, has annexed to frequent violations of his laws**: William Andrus Alcott, *The Physiology of Marriage* (J. P. Jewett & Co., 1856), 215, 67.

111. **Woloson reports that as early as the 1830s**: For the citations in this paragraph and the next, see chapter 2 in Woloson, esp. 61 ff.

112. **In a 2009 paper for the *International Journal of Obesity***: Mark B. Cope and David B. Allison, "White Hat Bias: Examples of Its Presence in Obesity Research and a Call for Renewed Commitment to Faithfulness in Research Reporting," *International Journal of Obesity* 34.1 (2009): 84–88.

112. **This so-called fact is based on a single 2001 study**: David S. Ludwig, Karen E. Peterson, and Steven L. Gortmaker, "Relation Between Consumption of Sugar-Sweetened Drinks and Childhood Obesity: A Prospective, Observational Analysis," *The Lancet* 357.9255 (2001): 505–8.

114. **wrote an entire column defending Allison's research and his credentials**: David Katz, "Research Funding: When Is the Money Dirty?" June 13, 2014, http://www.huffingtonpost. com/david-katz-md/research-funding-when-is-_b_5493613.html.

CHAPTER 5

120. **Exceptions are made for super-sweaty people like competitive athletes, foundry workers, and firefighters**: AHA, "Frequently Asked Questions (FAQs) About Sodium," http:// www.heart.org/HEARTORG/GettingHealthy/NutritionCenter/HealthyEating/Frequently-Asked-Questions-FAQs-About-Sodium_UCM_306840_Article.jsp.

120. **The AHA say that excess salt intake will result in between 500,000 and 1.2 million preventable deaths**: Ibid.

121. **Consider an eating plan advocated by American physician and diet guru John McDougall**: "Salt: The Scapegoat for the Western Diet," *McDougall Newsletter,* August 2008, https://www.drmcdougall.com/misc/2008nl/aug/salt.htm.

121. **told Americans to consume no more than 3 grams of salt per day**: United States, Congress, Senate, Select Committee on Nutrition and Human Needs, *Diet Related to Killer Diseases: Hearings before the Select Committee on Nutrition and Human Needs of the United States Senate, Ninety-Fifth Congress, first session* (Washington: U.S. Government Printing Office, 1977), 157.

122. **In a 2013 commentary for the journal** *Epidemiology*: Jiang He and Tanika Kelly, "Commentary: Sodium and Blood Pressure: Never Too Late to Reduce Dietary Intake," *Epidemiology* 24.3 (2013): 419–20.

123. **The origin of the quote is actually a 1956 anthology**: Arthur Ruskin, *Classics in Arterial Hypertension* (C. C. Thomas, 1956), xi ff.

123. **When I checked the original, the only passage that could be construed as referring to high blood pressure**: See Paul U. Unschuld, and Hermann Tessenow, *Huang Di Nei Jing Su Wen: An Annotated Translation of Huang Di's Inner Classic–Basic Questions: 2 volumes* (University of California Press, 2011), 559, n. 98. Here, Wang Bing says that salt is employed for treating [excessive fire qi]. In traditional Chinese medicine, high blood pressure is often understood as excess "yang qi" or "fire qi." This is a mistake—there are really no good analogues for many modern concepts in TCM, and blood pressure really doesn't exist in TCM. The other places where salt might be connected to high blood pressure are 10-70-6 (是 故 多 食 鹹 則 脈 凝 泣) and 12-80-2 (鹽 者 勝 血). Neither fits the bill. As Paul Unschuld wrote in an e-mail to me: "To trace a relationship between high blood pressure and the consumption of salt to the Suwen—nice fantasy, far off from historical reality. The simple fact to be taken into account is: since there was no concept of 'blood pressure,' there could not be a concept of 'increased blood pressure.'"

123. **bathing in dog feces**: Donald Harper, *Early Chinese Medical Literature: The Mawangdui Medical Manuscripts* (London: Kegan Paul International, 1998), 171.

124. **Salt also had a distinguished history in medicine**: For the definitive history of salt, see Mark Kurlansky, *Salt: A World History* (Walker and Company, 2002).

125. **heaviness of mind**: Ibid., 120.

125. **The first study to suggest salt's darker side came in 1904**: Ambard Beaujard, "Causes de l'hypertension artérielles," *Arch Gén Méd* 1 (1904): 520–33.

125. **A diet which is reasonably satisfying and at the same time sufficiently poor in salt is not so easy to arrange**: Frederick M. Allen, "Arterial Hypertension," *Journal of the American Medical Association* 74.10 (1920): 652–55, 654.

125. **judged the evidence inconclusive**: See, for instance, James G. O'Hare and William G. Walker, "Observations on Salt in Vascular Hypertension," *Archives of Internal Medicine* 32.2 (1923): 283–97.

125. **A massive, best-selling early-twentieth-century compendium of medical knowledge called** *The Library of Health*: B. Frank Scholl, ed., *The Library of Health: Complete Guide to Prevention and Cure of Disease* (Historical Publishing: 1935).

125–6. **On June 12, 1944, the Associated Press reported that Walter Kempner of Duke University**: Howard W. Blakeslee, "Rice Diet Used to Fight High Blood Pressure," Associated Press, June 12, 1944.

126. **During his first few years in America, Kempner practiced English**: For Kempner's early history, including his use of alligators, see Barbara Newborg and Florence Nash, *Walter Kempner and the Rice Diet: Challenging Conventional Wisdom* (Carolina Academic Press, 2011).

127. **Five years later, he presented his results to the American Medical Association in Chicago**: See Philip Klemmer, Clarence E. Grim, and Friedrich C. Luft, "Who and What Drove

Walter Kempner? The Rice Diet Revisited," *Hypertension* 64.4 (2014): 684–88. See also E. Harvey Estes and Lauren Kerivan, "An Archaeologic Dig: A Rice-Fruit Diet Reverses ECG Changes in Hypertension," *Journal of Electrocardiology* (2014).

127. **which sounds bad until you compare his overall results with the typical 6-month life expectancy of patients**: Philip Klemmer, Clarence E. Grim, and Friedrich C. Luft, "Who and What Drove Walter Kempner? The Rice Diet Revisited," *Hypertension* 64.4 (2014): 684–88.

127. **Skeptics accused Kempner of falsifying dates**: Ibid.

128. **As soon as a physician named Lewis K. Dahl identified the secret of the Rice Diet in 1950**: Vincent P. Dole, Lewis K. Dahl, George C. Cotzias, Howard A. Eder, and Margaret E. Krebs, "Dietary Treatment of Hypertension. Clinical and Metabolic studies of Patients on the Rice-Fruit Diet," *Journal of Clinical Investigation* 29.9 (1950): 1189.

128. **After examining the fluctuations in blood pressure experienced by the patients, Dahl saw a clear correlation to sodium intake**: Ibid. In a subsequent study conducted in the same manner, Dahl concluded that patients on the Rice Diet lost weight thanks to the absence of protein, independent of calorie consumption, a conclusion that does not inspire great confidence in his other results: Vincent P. Dole, Lewis K. Dahl, Irving L. Schwartz, George C. Cotzias, Jørn H. Thaysen, and Cecilia Harris, "Dietary Treatment of Hypertension. III. The Effect of Protein on Appetite and Weight," *Journal of Clinical Investigation* 32.2 (1953).

128. **In 1954 he analyzed surveys of "truly primitive human races"**: Lewis K. Dahl and R. A. Love, "Evidence for Relationship Between Sodium (Chloride) Intake and Human Essential Hypertension," *Archives of Internal Medicine* 94.4 (1954): 525–31.

129. **Nature is their only midwife**: Benjamin Rush, *Medical Inquiries and Observations*, *Vol. I,* Second Edition (Philadelphia, 1805), 10.

129. **till they were instructed to [use salt] by the Europeans**: Ibid., 8.

129. **This is not entirely true—some North American indigenous peoples actually had salt deities**: See Kurlansky, *Salt*, 202.

130. **We have evidence which suggests that among societies chronically on a high salt diet**: United States, Congress, Senate, Select Committee on Nutrition and Human Needs, *Hearings, Reports and Prints of the Senate Select Committee on Nutrition and Human Needs* (U.S. Government Printing Office, 1969), 3995.

130. **Baby Food Salt May Be Harmful, Researcher Says**: "Baby Food Salt May Be Harmful, Researcher Says," *Times Record,* April 28, 1970.

130. **A 1970 National Academy of Sciences committee declared there was "no evidence"**: Ronald Bayer, David Merritt Johns, and Sandro Galea, "Salt and Public Health: Contested Science and the Challenge of Evidence-Based Decision Making," *Health Affairs* 31.12 (2012): 2738–46.

130. **In 1977 Baker/Beech-Nut revealed a new line of "natural baby foods" free of added salt**: Frank Zell, "Baby Foods Change Seasonings—Sugar, Salt," *Chicago Tribune*, February 3, 1971. Cited in Bayer, et al.

131. **In the words of a 1978 article from the *American Journal of Clinical Nutrition***: R. J. Contreras, "Salt Taste and Disease," *American Journal of Clinical Nutrition* 31.6 (1978): 1088–97.

132. **Lewis Dahl himself compared the relationship between cigarette smoking and cancer**: Lewis K. Dahl, Martha Heine, George Leitl, and Lorraine Tassinari, "Hypertension and

Death from Consumption of Processed Baby Foods by Rats," *Experimental Biology and Medicine* 133.4 (1970): 1405–8.

132. **British newspapers uncovered industry funded studies of salt and political manipulation**: Bayer, et al.

132. **The food industry has everything to gain from keeping the controversy alive**: Fiona Godlee, "The Food Industry Fights for Salt," *BMJ* 312.7041 (1996): 1239–40.

133. **the results argue against reduction of dietary sodium**: Suzanne Oparil, "Low Sodium Intake—Cardiovascular Health Benefit or Risk?," *New England Journal of Medicine* 371.7 (2014): 677–79.

133. **Although Dr. Oparil reports receiving grants or fees from companies**: Marion Nestle, "It's salt war time again: new research, arguments over public health recommendations, and issues of conflicts of interest," Foodpolitics.com, August 14, 2014.

133. **The results were first discussed in 1988, in the *British Medical Journal***: P. Pietinen, U. Uusitalo, A. Nissinen, and Intersalt Cooperative Research Group, "Intersalt: An International Study of Electrolyte Excretion and Blood Pressure, Results for 24 Hour Urinary Sodium and Potassium Excretion," *BMJ: British Medical Journal* (1988).

134. **evangelical fervor**: J. D. Swales, "Salt Saga Continued," *BMJ: British Medical Journal* 297.6644 (1988): 307.

134. **Gary Taubes brought that dissent to light**: Gary Taubes, "The (Political) Science of Salt," *Science*, August 14, 1998.

135. **salt-induced hypertension is not attributable to intravascular fluid expansion**: Irene Gavras and Haralambos Gavras, "'Volume-Expanded' Hypertension: The Effect of Fluid Overload and the Role of the Sympathetic Nervous System in Salt-Dependent Hypertension," *Journal of Hypertension* 30.4 (2012): 655–59.

135. **In an exhaustive 2012 history of the salt wars**: Ronald Bayer, David Merritt Johns, and Sandro Galea, "Salt and Public Health: Contested Science and the Challenge of Evidence-Based Decision Making," *Health Affairs* 31.12 (2012): 2738–46.

135. **surprisingly little rationale**: Aaron Carroll, "Dash of Salt Does No Harm, Extremes Are the Enemy," *New York Times*, August 26, 2014.

135. **the CDC recommends that all adults age fifty-one or older and all African Americans reduce sodium intake to 1,500 mg**: "Most Americans Should Consume Less Sodium," accessed October 28, 2014, http://www.cdc.gov/salt.

135. **no evidence in favor of treating African Americans or the elderly any differently**: IOM, "Sodium Intake in Populations: Assessment of Evidence," May 2013, http://www.iom.edu/~/media/Files/Report%20Files/2013/Sodium-Intake-Populations/SodiumIntakeinPopulations_RB.pdf.

136. **And they remain in place despite a 2014 Canadian study**: Martin O'Donnell, Andrew Mente, Sumathy Rangarajan, Matthew J. McQueen, Xingyu Wang, Lisheng Liu, Hou Yan, et al., "Urinary Sodium and Potassium Excretion, Mortality, and Cardiovascular Events," *New England Journal of Medicine* 371.7 (2014): 612–23.

136. **well below the global average of 3,950 mg**: Lenny Berstein, "Salt Intake Is Too High in 181 of 187 Countries around the World," *Washington Post*, August 14, 2014.

137. **$8 million that Kempner donated to the medical center**: AP, "Faculty Doctor Donates $8M to Duke," October 8, 1997.

137. **$30 million annually to the local economy**: Tim Gray, "Heavy Industry," *Business North Carolina,* July 2006.

137. **Newspapers across the nation picked up a shocking story of abuse and brainwashing that had first come to light in 1993**: AP, "Report: Rice Diet Doctor Admitted to Whippings in Depositions," October 19, 1997.

137. **former patient Rebecca Reynolds**: Name changed at the request of the subject.

137. **virtual sex slave/servant**: Bob Ellinger, "Case against Duke Rice Diet King Continues Despite Roadblocks," *Duke Chronicle,* October 23, 1997.

138. **I was crying because I thought I was bad, deserved to be whipped**: Ibid.

138. **Reynolds was not alone in her worship**: The details provided about Kempner and the Kreis come from a detailed article published in the Charlotte *News Observer*: Chris O'Brien, Wendy Howes, "Suit Reveals Kempner's Guarded Private Life," October 19, 1997.

139. **Kempner refused to use control groups**: Klemmer, "Who and What Drove Walter Kempner?," and also Newborg, *Walter Kempner and the Rice Diet.*

140. **For a good look at what happened to Fat City visitors, there is no better book than *Fat Like Us***: Jean Renfro Anspaugh, *Fat Like Us* (Generation Books, 2001). All references in "The Low Salt Cult" are taken from Renfro.

143. **Jeffrey Steingarten wrote an essay in 1990 complaining about the hysterical anti-salt environment in America**: "Salt," in Jeffrey Steingarten, *The Man Who Ate Everything* (New York: Random House LLC, 2011).

143. **The food tastes mainly of herbs, spices, garlic, and onions**: Ibid., 197.

144. **Tim Carman decided to try reducing his salt to 1,500 mg**: Tim Carman, "How Hard Is It to Reduce Your Salt?," *Washington Post,* February 15, 2011.

144. **generally required considerable efforts**: Rod S. Taylor, Kate E. Ashton, Tiffany Moxham, Lee Hooper, and Shah Ebrahim, "Reduced Dietary Salt for the Prevention of Cardiovascular Disease: A Meta-Analysis of Randomized Controlled Trials (Cochrane Reviews)," *American Journal of Hypertension* 24.8 (2011): 843–53.

144. **Many of us have developed a preference for salty flavours**: Consensus Action on Salt, "How to eat less salt," http://www.actiononsalt.org.uk/less/Reducing%20Intake/79609.html.

145. **Taste food as it really should taste**: http://www.actiononsalt.org.uk/resources/Postcard/88012.pdf.

145. **Change your salty ways**: http://www.heart.org/HEARTORG/GettingHealthy/NutritionCenter/HealthyEating/Sodium-Swap-Change-Your-Salty-Ways-in-21-Days-Infographic_UCM_455060_SubHomePage.jsp.

145. **slinks into soups and sandwiches**: AHA, "How to Track Your Sodium," http://www.heart.org/HEARTORG/Conditions/More/MyHeartandStrokeNews/How-to-Track-Your-Sodium_UCM_449547_Article.jsp?appName=MobileApp.

145. **Even after reducing the sodium content of all U.S. foods by 10 percent**: Matthieu Maillot, Pablo Monsivais, and Adam Drewnowski, "Food Pattern Modeling Shows That the 2010 Dietary Guidelines for Sodium and Potassium Cannot Be Met Simultaneously," *Nutrition Research* 33.3 (2013): 188–94.

146. **Hormel's "Sin Free" line**: http://www.hormelhealthlabs.com/2colTemplate_product.aspx?page=CO_SinFree&cond_id=132&cat_id=136.

146. **"Guiltless Gourmet" unsalted potato chips**: http://www.guiltlessgourmet.com.

146. **to eat with pleasure is something I will never experience**: Renfro, *Fat Like Us*, 240.

CHAPTER 6

147. **they endorsed a variety of dubious dietary supplements**: Robert Ford Campany, *To Live as Long as Heaven and Earth: A Translation and Study of Ge Hong's Traditions of Divine Transcendents* (University of California Press, 2002).

147. **It is prepared by taking some blood from the chick**: Ibid., 289.

148. **The recipe**: Dave Asprey, "Recipe: How to Make Your Coffee Bulletproof" . . . And Your Morning Too," accessed October 28, 2014, https://www.bulletproofexec.com/how-to-make-your-coffee-bulletproof-and-your-morning-too.

148. **clean coffee actually fights cancer**: Once Bulletproof® became a diet book, the shameful, exploitative claim about fighting cancer was scrubbed from Asprey's website. See the archived page: http://web.archive.org/web/20140701034518/https://www.bulletproofexec.com/how-to-make-your-coffee-bulletproof-and-your-morning-too.

148. **"lose 100 pounds without using exercise" and "upgrade your IQ by more than 12 points"**: https://www.bulletproofexec.com.

149. **According to *Men's Health* magazine**: Jonny Bowden, "The Ten Best Foods You Aren't Eating," http://www.menshealth.com/mhlists/best_healthy_foods/Goji_Berries.php.

150. **In *The Fruit Hunters*, journalist Adam Leith Gollner documents how a man named Earl Mindell**: Adam Leith Gollner, *The Fruit Hunters: A Story of Nature, Adventure, Commerce, and Obsession* (New York: Simon and Schuster, 2013). Mindell's story is on p. 164.

150. **his books, including *Earl Mindell's Soy Miracle* and *The Vitamin Bible*, have sold millions of copies**: James A. Lowell, "An Irreverent Look at the Vitamin Bible and Its Author (Earl Mindell)," Nutrition Forum, June 1986, http://www.quackwatch.com/04Consumer Education/NegativeBR/vbible.html.

150. **How long would you like to live, asks Mindell**: Cited in Leith, 164.

151. **As reported in *Men's Journal***: Adam Hadhazy, "Should You Be Drinking Bulletproof Coffee?" *Men's Journal*, January 28, 2014.

152. **The scare over carrageenan has been based on the work and activism of one scientist**: For an excellent history of carrageenan, see Duika Burges Watson, "Public health and carrageenan regulation: a review and analysis," *Nineteenth International Seaweed Symposium* (Springer Netherlands, 2009), 55–63. Yes, the International Seaweed Symposium.

153. **She has now shifted her focus to connecting carrageenan with irritable bowel syndrome and diabetes**: S. Bhattacharyya, I. O-Sullivan, S. Katyal, T. Unterman, and J. K. Tobacman, "Exposure to the Common Food Additive Carrageenan Leads to Glucose Intolerance, Insulin Resistance and Inhibition of Insulin Signalling in HepG2 Cells and C57BL/6J Mice," *Diabetologia* 55.1 (2012): 194–203.

153. **The Committee concluded that the use of carrageenan in infant formula or formula for special medical purposes**: Joint FAO/WHO Expert Committee on Food Additives, "Summary and Conclusions," July 2, 2014, http://www.who.int/foodsafety/publications/Summary79.pdf?ua=1.

153. **In August 2014, the "Food Babe" and her "Food Babe Army" pressured White-Wave Foods**: Vani Hari, "BREAKING: Major Company Removing Controversial Ingredient Carrageenan Because of You!," Foodbabe.com, August 19, 2014.

154. **most, if not all, of the degenerative diseases that afflict us**: http://www.forksoverknives.com/synopsis.

155. **"Is everything we eat associated with cancer?"**: Jonathan D. Schoenfeld and John P. A. Ioannidis., "Is Everything We Eat Associated with Cancer? A Systematic Cookbook Review," *American Journal of Clinical Nutrition* 97.1 (2013): 127–34.

156. **as Vibram USA did in 2014, a lawsuit they settled for $3.75 million**: Emily Thomas, "Vibram, 'Barefoot Running Shoe' Company, Settles Multi-Million Dollar Lawsuit," Huffingtonpost.com, May 13, 2014.

157. **honor a wisdom in evolution**: "Why Vaccines Aren't Paleo," GreenMedInfo.com, February 23, 2014, http://www.greenmedinfo.com/blog/why-vaccines-arent-paleo.

157. **admits he decided not to vaccinate his nine-month-old daughter**: "We haven't given Sylvie any vaccinations at all. She's nine months old now . . . " From transcript of a podcast, Chris Kresser, "RHR: CoQ10, Vaccination, and Natural Treatment for Migraines," May 2, 2012.

157. **Mothers in my study describe their efforts to protect their children's health in ways they see as making vaccines unnecessary**: Jennifer Reich, "Neo-Liberal Mothering and Vaccine Refusal," September 2, 2014, http://gendersociety.wordpress.com/2014/09/02/neoliberal-mothering-and-vaccine-refusal.

158. **Horror in the Nursery**: Judith Crist, "Horror in the Nursery," *Collier's* 27 (1948): 22–23.

158. **book burning later that year in Spencer, West Virginia**: Jacqui Shine, "The Great Comic Book Conflagration," Laphamsquarterly.org, August 12, 2014.

158. **Christopher Ferguson of Texas A&M leading the way in arguing that moral panic**: See, for instance: Christopher J. Ferguson, "The School Shooting/Violent Video Game Link: Causal Relationship or Moral Panic?," *Journal of Investigative Psychology and Offender Profiling* 5.1–2 (2008): 25–37.

160. **they are far *less* obsessed with the healthfulness of what they eat**: Paul Rozin, Claude Fischler, Sumio Imada, Allison Sarubin, and Amy Wrzesniewski. "Attitudes to Food and the Role of Food in Life in the USA, Japan, Flemish Belgium and France: Possible Implications for the Diet–Health Debate," *Appetite* 33.2 (1999): 163–80.

160. **in the majority of cases *dieting results in more weight gain than doing nothing at all***: Evelyn Tribole, "Warning: Dieting Increases Your Risk of Gaining MORE Weight (An Update)," Intuitiveeating.com, accessed October 28, 2014.

160. **One study of Finnish twins found that, independent of genetics**: K. H. Pietiläinen, S. E. Saarni, J. Kaprio, and A. Rissanen, "Does Dieting Make You Fat?; A Twin Study," *International Journal of Obesity* 36.3 (2011): 456–64.

160. **converted the stroll into exercise and food into calories**: For this and the following quotes, see Max Horkheimer and Theodor W. Adorno, *Dialectic of Enlightenment: Philosophical Fragments*, E. Jephcott, translator (Stanford: 2002), 195–96.

161. ***eating in the fourth dimension***: Jay Olshansky came up with this phrase in a conversation with me and generously allowed me to use it. With attribution, of course!

Further Reading

If you want to learn more about the cultural significance of dietary practices, anthropologist Mary Douglas's *Purity and Danger* is a must-read classic. For a detailed survey of food taboos and their meaning, check out Frederick Simoons's *Eat Not This Flesh*. On the history of American eating, Harvey Levenstein has three great books: *Revolution at the Table*, *Paradox of Plenty*, and *Fear of Food*.

If you're more of a diet and health claims skeptic, Tim Caufield's *The Cure for Everything* does a nice job sorting hyperbole from sound science. For "alternative" medicine specifically, try Paul Offit's *Do You Believe In Magic?* And on the nefarious influence of the pharmaceutical industry, there's nothing better than Ben Goldacre's *Bad Pharma*.

Irritated by nutrition gurus? Wonder how they live with themselves? James Hamblin's "This Is Your Brain on Gluten" (theatlantic.com) and Michael Specter's "The Operator" (newyorker.com) are amazing snapshots of David Perlmutter and Mehmet Oz, respectively.

For those who want to lose weight, Brian Wansink's *Mindless Eating* and Yoni Freedhoff's *The Diet Fix* offer sensible guidance that doesn't demonize food or promise miracles.

Finally, two trustworthy blogs in a sea of unreliable nonsense:

The Incidental Economist: primary focus on health care, run by statistician Austin Frankt and pediatrician Aaron Carroll. theincidentaleconomist.com

Science-Based Medicine: skeptical evaluations of medical claims and treatments, founded by neurologist Steven Novella. (Novella's 2011 appearance on Dr. Oz is amazing.) sciencebasedmedicine.org

Index